DIALYSIS CHAMPIONS OF THE NEW-ERA THRU THE
KNOWLEDGE POWER
OF "EVIDENCE-BASED PRACTICE RESEARCH"

DIALYSIS CHAMPIONS OF THE NEW-ERA THRU THE KNOWLEDGE POWER OF "EVIDENCE-BASED PRACTICE RESEARCH"

ROSEMARIE ZULETA MSN, BSN, CNN

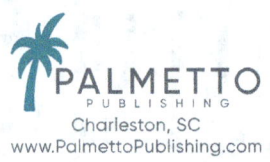
Charleston, SC
www.PalmettoPublishing.com

Dialysis Champions of the New-Era
Thru the Knowledge Power of "Evidence-Based Practice Research"
Copyright © 2023 by Rosemarie Zuleta MSN, BSN, CNN

All rights reserved
No portion of this book may be reproduced, stored in a retrieval system, or transmitted in any form by any means–electronic, mechanical, photocopy, recording, or other– except for brief quotations in printed reviews, without prior permission of the author.

First Edition

Hardcover ISBN: 979-8-8229-2446-8
Paperback ISBN: 979-8-8229-2416-1

Dedication

This project is dedicated to my family, who have supported me throughout my writing journey. Specifically, my mother who has put up with my long hours away from the family and has taken on more responsibilities, allowing me the time and motivation to complete my degree and achieve my goals.

ACKNOWLEDGMENT

I am humbled and glad for the opportunity to offer my sincere gratitude to everyone who helped create and publish my book, "Dialysis Champion of the New Era Thru the Knowledge Power of 'Evidence-Based Practice Research." First, I want to thank my family for their constant support and encouragement during this journey. Their compassion and understanding have been a continual motivation for me, allowing me to follow my passion and complete this book.

Secondly, I want to convey my heartfelt gratitude to my mentor, Alice Hellebrand, DNP, MSN, CNN, whose advice and knowledge have been priceless. Her intelligent input, constructive criticism, and steadfast faith in my talents have all played critical roles in the development of this book. Next, I extend my gratitude to the dialysis medical professionals, researchers, and specialists whose relentless work and revolutionary discoveries have paved the path for advances in patient care. Because of their passion and commitment, I have been able to investigate and comprehend the complexities of dialysis, enabling me to share this information with the rest of the world.

I thank my coworkers and friends for their help, encouragement, and insightful insights during the writing process. Their friendship and debates have enhanced the substance of this book and turned it into a joint effort. Plus, all their enthusiasm and participation in the topic drive writers like myself to strive for perfection. Their ideas and passion are greatly appreciated.

Finally, I thank the editing team and publishing professionals who worked tirelessly to turn my manuscript into a published work. Their attention to detail, experience, and devotion have all contributed to the success of this work. Their dedication to establishing a culture of knowledge and learning has aided in the development of the evidence-based approach provided in this book.

Thank you for being a part of this fantastic adventure.

Sincerely,

Rosemarie Zuleta, MSN, BSN, CNN

07/17/2023

ABOUT THE AUTHOR

My journey to becoming an author of a dialysis book did not begin overnight. I started my career in nursing at Chinatown Dialysis Center in the US in 2009. In the same way that most Filipino nurses do, I arrived in the US as a qualified nurse who needed to explore in Dialysis Nursing Program to be eligible to become an experienced Dialysis US nurse. The first half of a year was a rough go for me. It was challenging to adjust to a new position and setting, and it was unpleasant to have to confine your practice to that context. Later, I went to work for a Dialysis healthcare company which is Dialyze Direct until in present time, until I was offered my current position. Because there are usually other Filipino coworkers in whatever department I have worked in, I have always felt like an integral part of the team.

In my opinion, renal nursing is a dynamic field with plenty of room for growth, improvement and its share of challenges. Hospitals have several care units, such as those for chronic, acute, and peritoneal patients. Throughout my career in renal nursing, I have taken advantage of many secondment possibilities (working temporarily somewhere with the approval of my management and the understanding that my original job would be "reserved" for me upon completion). In my nursing career, I have "rotated" between acute dialysis and renal ward nursing, renal vascular access coordination, renal research nursing, and leadership responsibilities in outpatient dialysis. At the facility where I work, there are subspecialist nursing positions for home therapies, renal anemia, quick assessment, outpatient day cases, and conservative management.

I engage with various CKD patients daily and collaborate closely with their primary care physicians and renal consultants. I work with them to organize medication adjustments and requests for further evaluations. This was a brand-new capability for me, and it was also a previously identified weakness. Therefore, I have focused on developing my capacity for clear and compelling expression via writing and other forms of communication. I asked for input from our consultants on how well I communicated with my primary care colleagues through letters and texts. The uncertainty surrounding advanced nursing practice is another difficult aspect of my job. Given that patients on chronic dialysis are often stable and their clinical issues are very prevalent, this may seem ironic and atypical for a conventional renal outpatient treatment. Renal dialysis nursing can be demanding and rewarding; therefore, it is critical to identify these issues and act quickly.

One of my most outstanding achievements was authoring and publishing my first book on dialysis. In my book, I wanted to show that there is life to be had and that it can be good, even while on dialysis. I drew on my extensive medical training and experience in dialysis departments to address common concerns about the treatment, including how it may affect the patient's ability to eat normally, engage in physical activity, and participate in social events. I have described the dialysis process in detail, including the many treatment options available, the benefits and drawbacks of a kidney transplant, and the potential adverse reactions. Since dialysis impacts the whole family, I have shared the humor, fortitude, and successes of families who have successfully confronted the obstacles of dialysis, offering genuine insights into how relatives may manage and prosper together. The result is a motivational, actionable handbook that will teach dialysis patients and their loved ones how to deal with the challenges of dialysis, face life without fear, and make the most of each day.

As we advance into the future, I want to inspire other aspiring nurses to venture into the dialysis field and become a reliable advocates for my dialysis patients. My main responsibility as a dialysis advocate would be to inform newly diagnosed patients of their choices for dialysis therapy, including home hemodialysis and outpatient dialysis mode, as well as other methods of kidney care. Because most patients do not have easy access to their legislators in Congress, I want to ensure that every patient's voice is heard and that all dialysis patients have the tools to take control of their health. I want to be the first point of contact for those coping with renal illness, providing vital information and emotional support.

I want to aid those dealing with renal illness adjust to their potentially dialysis-related new normal. Moreover, as an advocate, I want to provide an entry point for dialysis patients to learn about what is occurring in their bodies, how to manage their health, and what treatment options are available if they need to begin dialysis or contemplate a transplant throughout this life-altering journey. Patients with kidney illnesses will greatly benefit from having someone guide them through getting ready for dialysis.

Page Blank Intentionally

PREFACE

This book has been written to address the needs of the health care professionals belonging to the Nephrology department. It is written to assist all such professionals in understanding the principles and applications of the technologies and information known currently. The text is written in a simple and easy-to-understand language, making it accessible to everyone with an average or higher understanding of English. In this regard, you need not be equipped with prior advanced knowledge. This book is suitable for all healthcare professionals and undergraduate and postgraduate students undergoing studies, examinations, or training in nephrology. All clinical aspects of information, supervision, training, and other related elements have been covered in this book related to the nephrology department.

The book is written for all those involved in kidney patients' treatment, diagnosis, and care. Those looking to pursue a career in this field, including healthcare professionals, doctors, nurses, and all staff associated with the nephrology department, will find this book helpful. Those with a background in medicine or related field will find this resource valuable in studying the broad knowledge available. The book summarizes the unique challenges healthcare professionals and patients face in managing and treating various forms of kidney disease. It also helps create awareness about the multiple complexities in this field, besides preparing people to make informed decisions about ensuring good kidney health.

The treatment of kidney diseases has undergone numerous changes in the last decade or so. New treatment options that are better in place to treat and assist have emerged, while technology has revolutionized the treatment process. Old ideas need to be updated, while the flaws in practice need to be identified and addressed. Overcoming the common mistakes many healthcare professionals unknowingly commit is important as it will improve patient outcomes and treatment, benefiting patients and society.

Writing the book was a formidable task, but completed with the tiring efforts of the writer. Her knowledge, experience, skills, and training have contributed to this book, which will be a valuable resource. The clarity of the text will make it easier for you to understand and apply the principles discussed in this book.

TABLE OF CONTENTS

Acknowledgment i
About the Author iii
Preface vii

Chapter 1: Significance of a Functional Kidney to Acute/Chronic
        Kidney Failure. 1
Chapter 2: Participating in the Dialysis 25
Chapter 3: Root Causes of the Dialysis Problems. 39
Chapter 4: Dialysis-Related Matters 59
Chapter 5: Inflammation and Pain 81
Chapter 6: Clotting Problems and DVT in the Circulatory System . . 97
Chapter 7: Dialysate Temperature and pH Balance. 115
Chapter 8: Stroke and HTN 131
Chapter 9: Lab values involved in Dialysis and Assessment Process . .147
Chapter 10: Common Cause of Death among the Dialysis Patients . .167
Chapter 11: Dialyzable Medications 181
Chapter 12: Dialysis Patients Battling with Mental Health Issues . . .195
Chapter 13: Delving more into Quality Assessment and Performance
        Improvement on ESRD. 211
Chapter 14: Transforming Lives through Kidney Transplant 219
Chapter 15: Benefits of Medicare coverage for End Stage Renal
        Disease (ESRD) people .233
Chapter 16: Healthy Lifestyle. 243
Chapter 17: How to Become an Effective Nurse 257
Chapter 18: Life Stories of an R.N. Treating Dialysis Patient. 263

Chapter 19: NxStage Home Hemodialysis 267
Chapter 20: The Future of Your Health is in Your Hands and
            Evolving Modern Dialysis Technology is around the
            Corner 275

Index 281

CHAPTER ONE:
SIGNIFICANCE OF A FUNCTIONAL KIDNEY TO ACUTE/CHRONIC KIDNEY FAILURE

The essential function of the kidney

First, let us talk about the kidneys; the kidneys are two bean-shaped organs located on either side of the spine, beneath your ribs, and behind your abdomen. Each kidney is 4 to 5 inches long and about the size of a huge hand. Most people realize that the kidneys' primary function is to remove waste from the body by washing it away with urine.

However, many individuals are unaware that kidneys do other wonderful functions for which they should be grateful.

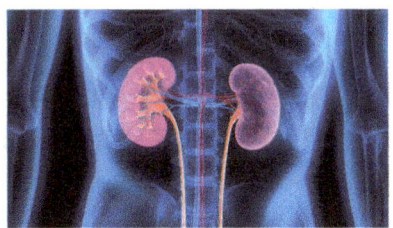

Here are a few essential functions of the kidney.

1. **Maintaining acid-base balance**

   The acids and bases in the human body are always in a delicate equilibrium, as reflected by the pH value. The normal blood pH ranges from 7.35 to 7.45. To keep the body in a healthy range, the kidneys expel acids and bases when there is an excess of them and store these compounds when the body is deficient. The pace at which your kidneys filter waste is known as the glomerular filtration rate (GFR). This GFR will be lower if your kidneys are injured. Your estimated glomerular filtration rate (eGFR) and various stages of damage are shown by blood testing. [1]

2. **Blood pressure maintenance**

   Renin is an enzyme produced by the kidneys. Renin transforms angiotensinogen generated in the liver into angiotensin I, which is then turned into angiotensin II in the lungs. Angiotensin II constricts blood vessels, causing blood pressure to rise. When one's blood pressure is excessively high, the kidneys generate more urine to decrease the Volume of liquid circulating in the body and somewhat compensate for the high blood pressure.

3. **Osmolality regulation**

   The kidneys aid in the maintenance of the body's water and salt levels. The hypothalamus, which connects directly with the posterior pituitary gland, detects any considerable increase in plasma osmolality. When osmolality rises, the gland secretes antidiuretic hormone (ADH), which stimulates water reabsorption by the

---

[1] https://www.webmd.com/a-to-z-guides/what-to-know-about-stages-chronic-kidney-disease

kidney and increases urine concentration. The two components work together to restore normal plasma osmolality levels.[2]

4. **Vitamin D activation**

It produces the hormones calcitriol and erythropoietin. Calcitriol is a kind of vitamin D that aids in calcium absorption. The kidneys convert Calcifediol into Calcitriol, the active form of vitamin D. Calcitriol circulates in the blood. It regulates calcium and phosphate balance in the body, which is necessary for proper bone formation. Erythropoietin is a hormone that aids in producing red blood cells in the body.

Calcitonin is another hormone secreted by the thyroid gland, which adapts to the function of the PTH hormone in response to hypocalcemia. This hormone counteracts hypercalcemia and prevents osteoclasts' activity. It stimulates the calcium and phosphates deposit to bones.

5. **Removing toxins and waste from the body**

The kidneys filter out water-soluble waste products and poisons, washing them out of the body with urine. That is why kidney failure swiftly leads to severe intoxication, as the body's waste products accumulate and impede its functions.

6. **Measuring function**

Various computations and procedures are used to attempt to measure renal function. Renal clearance is the Volume of plasma

---

2 https://pubmed.ncbi.nlm.nih.gov/15453232/#:~:text=The%20kidneys%2C%20in%20concert%20with,differ%20within%20each%20nephron%20segment.

from which a drug is entirely removed from the blood per unit of time. The filtration fraction is the quantity of plasma filtered via the kidney. This can be defined using the equation. The kidney is a highly complicated organ, and mathematical modeling has been used to understand better renal function at multiple scales, including fluid uptake and secretion.

Hormones That Kidneys Produce to Help the Body's Homeostasis

They also play crucial roles in maintaining homeostasis in the body, such as regulating acid-base balance, electrolyte concentration, blood pressure management, and hormone secretion. Kidney failure creates a major and perhaps fatal disruption in the body's equilibrium. These complications include weakness, shortness of breath, extensive swelling (edema), metabolic acidosis, and cardiac rhythms.

The kidneys produce two essential hormones that help in homeostasis: erythropoietin and renin. Erythropoietin increases red blood cell synthesis in the bone marrow. This occurs due to these cells' natural turnover rates (life spans) and in reaction to cellular Hypoxia, which occurs when tissues do not receive enough Oxygen. Renin is a hormone and an enzyme commonly known as Angiotensinogenase. It is used to aid in synthesizing Angiotensin II, which has numerous effects on the body and eventually leads to elevated blood pressure. [3]

---

3   https://www.ncbi.nlm.nih.gov/books/NBK536997/#:~:text=Erythropoietin%20(EPO)%20is%20a%20glycoprotein,greater%20the%20production%20of%20EPO.

How do the Different Foods Good for Kidneys Compare

The kidneys are tiny organs in the lower abdomen crucial to the body's general health. While some foods generally maintain a healthy kidney, some may be harmful. So, it is essential to consume the right foods. A kidney-healthy eating plan can help the kidneys work properly and shield them from harm.

Blueberries

Blueberries are extremely nutritious since they include vitamin C, fiber, and antioxidants. They can reverse some of the problems resulting from CKD by reducing inflammation and supporting bone health.

Onions

Onions, members of the same family as garlic, provide another fantastic salt-free flavoring option (bonus points if you sauté them in olive oil). Additionally, onions include essential nutrients like manganese, copper, and vitamins B6 and C. They also have organic Sulphur compounds that can lower your risk of high blood pressure, stroke, and heart disease, and quercetin, which can help your body fight cancer.

Garlic

An active ingredient in garlic that helps to safeguard kidney health just as well as prescription medicine. (Colman, n.d.) garlic should be on your list of the top foods for renal health.

Whole grains

Whole grains, including oats, barley, whole wheat, brown rice, and quinoa, are beneficial for digestive and general health since they include a wealth of vitamins, minerals, and fiber. Choose buckwheat or bulgur (cracked wheat) if you limit your mineral consumption because they contain less potassium, salt, and phosphorus than grains like quinoa and oats.

Red peppers

The well-known antioxidant vitamin C is abundant in red peppers. They are suitable for persons with kidney disease to eat because they contain less potassium than some other vegetables. Additionally, they have vitamin A, a substance necessary for healthy immune system operation.

People who wish to keep their kidneys healthy and those with advanced kidney disease must follow a kidney-friendly diet. This is known as a renal diet, ensuring wastes do not accumulate in the blood. This diet is essential for boosting kidney function and preventing further damage from happening.

A Brief Comparison of the Nutritional Foods in a Renal Diet

Experts have recommended restricting the following nutrients in your diet if you are diagnosed with kidney disease.

Sodium

Found in many foods and being an integral part of table salt, this nutrient must be restricted to less than 2,000 mg daily. The problem with damaged kidneys is that they cannot filter out sodium if taken in excess, which then causes the blood levels to rise.

Potassium

No doubt potassium is important for the body as it is required for playing many different roles in the human body. However, if there is an underlying kidney issue, its intake must be limited, or it would lead to high blood levels that are dangerous for the body. The recommended limit is less than 2,000 mg per day.

Phosphorus

Found in many foods as a mineral, its intake needs to be restricted to less than 2,000 mg per day as a diseased kidney cannot remove excess phosphorus leading to high levels.

Protein

This nutrient needs to be limited if you have kidney disease. The reason is that protein metabolism gives rise to waste products, and damaged kidneys cannot remove the waste.

You may include the following foods in your diet which are cauliflower, blueberries, sea bass, red grapes, onions, bell peppers, radish, turnips, egg whites, garlic, cabbage, skinless chicken, buckwheat, olive oil, bulgur, and pineapple. However, there is no need to worry about restricting the intake of these nutrients, as many other healthy options for taste buds are available that are low in the nutrients mentioned above.

The outlook is always cheerful when following a renal diet, as many delicious foods can be consumed and made a part of a kidney-friendly diet plan.

The Role of Amount of Water in Keeping Kidneys Healthy

Drinking the right amount of water is imperative to keeping kidneys healthy. The most common notion is that an individual must drink at least eight glasses of water. However, the actual intake required varies from person to person. Other factors that impact the quantity of water needed are age, frequency of exercise, climate, pregnancy, breastfeeding, and illness. Water aids the kidneys in removing waste from the blood via urine. Water is also required to open the blood vessels so that they can travel to the kidney and deliver essential nutrients. Dehydration causes the kidneys not to function properly. Mild dehydration will make you tired and impair the functions of the different parts of the body. However, severe dehydration will cause damage to the kidneys. So, drink plenty of water, especially if you live in a place with a warm temperature.

As mentioned above, water intake depends on factors, like age and climate. The U.S.; dietary guidelines 2015-2020 did not recommend any specific quantity of water to be consumed. The U.K.'s NHS recommends 6 to 8 glasses of water every day. This also includes the water in the food. However, this amount is only suitable if you live in a temperate climate. You must drink more if you live in a country with a hotter climate.

Recommended Amount of Water Intake in Healthy Pediatric, Adulthood, and Geriatric Population

Infants

Plain water is not recommended for infants. According to the center for disease control (CDC), infants need to be given additional water in a bottle if the weather is hot, but still, the primary source of fluids should either be breast milk or formula.

Children after one year

After passing the age of 12 months, children need to be educated about drinking water. They should be encouraged to consume more water daily during warm weather. They should be encouraged to prefer water over sweetened drinks and juices.

Adults above 18 but below 30

The recommended amount of water intake is 3.7 liters for men and 2.7 liters for women. If a woman is pregnant, an extra 0.3 liters are required, while those who are breastfeeding need an additional 0.7 to 1.1 liters.

Older adults

Such individuals are at risk of dehydration. The increased risk is due to medications, health conditions, loss of muscle mass, and other factors, such as reduced kidney function.

There are many advantages of staying hydrated for older adults, such as fewer falls, avoiding constipation, and reduced risk of bladder cancer for older male adults.

Dehydration in older age contributes to urinary tract infections, kidney failure, and slower wound healing.

Maintaining the pH Balance and Hydration in Dialysis patients

Though staying hydrated is essential for those with CSK, it is also imperative that the patient avoid fluid overload, known as hypervolemia. A person on dialysis has kidneys that cannot maintain the right balance of fluids. Hence, limiting salt (sodium) and fluid intake becomes a crucial during dialysis treatment. Most dialysis patients are required to restrict fluid intake to 32 ounces per day. This precaution will help the body maintain fluid balance and ensure the removal of extra water.

Those who suffer from chronic kidney disease or end-stage kidney failure are susceptible to undergoing metabolic derangements, such as acid-base and electrolyte imbalances. Hence, maintaining the pH is necessary. Otherwise, the issue will materialize in the form of morbidity and mortality.

Patients affected by multiple acid-base and electrolytic derangements will find their condition worsening and becoming severe as chronic kidney disease progresses. The best option is optimal management though it can be pretty challenging. Study data are available to guide its management, and dialysis prescriptions are available.

The treatment demands a multi-pronged strategy to minimize the issue's severity. Dietary changes must be incorporated immediately, including restricting the patient to a renal diet. Dialysis prescriptions will further help in the treatment.

What is kidney disease?

Your kidneys gradually stop functioning correctly if you have chronic renal disease. The injury brings many phases of chronic kidney disease, which can permanently deteriorate over time.

Anyone can develop CKD; however, some people are more susceptible to it than others. People from South Asia and people of color are more likely to experience it, which is linked to aging. While elderly persons over 65 tend to have a stable illness, the condition often worsens when younger people have CKD. Chronic kidney disease has no known therapy or cure, although early detection and intervention can slow the progression of your condition. Many individuals with CKD have healthy, extended lives, but it is crucial to visit your doctor frequently to keep your illness under control.

Acute and Chronic Kidney Failure compared: Different Stages of Chronic Kidney Disease

Water, salts, and minerals like sodium, calcium, and potassium are balanced by your kidneys. Additionally, they produce hormones that help manufacture red blood cells, maintain bone density, and regulate blood pressure.

Through structures known as nephrons, your kidneys also remove extra fluid and waste from your body. Each nephron has a glomerulus, filters blood, and a tubule that separates waste from necessary blood components and returns them to circulation.

An abrupt onset marks acute kidney failure and can be potentially reversed with treatment. Chronic kidney failure, on the other hand, progresses slowly over at least three months. This condition potentially causes permanent kidney failure. The symptoms and treatment of both underlying conditions are different. While acute kidney failure is marked by sudden and severe symptoms that can be easily recognized, chronic kidney failure develops symptoms slowly and may be mistaken for other conditions. As mentioned earlier, acute kidney failure can be reversed once the underlying issue is addressed. In contrast, chronic kidney failure leads to permanent kidney failure and must be managed to ensure the kidneys continue functioning.

There are treatments available for chronic kidney disease which can help relieve symptoms and prevent the disease from worsening. Acute kidney failure can be treated by resolving the underlying condition. To determine if your kidneys are functioning well, the individual must undertake a simple panel of blood tests.

Stages of CKD

An important marker of renal function is creatinine, a waste product produced when muscles contract. When the kidneys function correctly, they eliminate creatinine from the blood; however, as renal function declines, blood creatinine levels increase. According to medical professionals, the severity of kidney disease is determined by the glomerular filtration rate (GFR), which is calculated using a person's age, gender, and serum creatinine level (identified through a blood test).

Here are some stages of kidney disease.

Stage 1

Standard or high GFR (GFR > 90 mL/min, less than 100)

The kidneys have undergone mild damage during this stage but still function normally.

Stage 2

Mild CKD (GFR = 60-89 mL/min)

Damage to the kidneys is more significant than in stage 1, but still, the kidneys are functioning well.

Stage 3

Moderate CKD (GFR = 30-59 mL/min)

Mild or severe loss results in a significant decrease in kidney functions and a significant decline in the removal of metabolic waste.

Stage 4

Severe CKD (GFR = 15-29 mL/min)

The severe loss suffered by the kidney and severe decline in kidney function. Metabolic waste is not being removed effectively.

Stage 5

End Stage CKD (GFR <15 mL/min)

Nearing or having completely failed kidneys and metabolic waste is not being removed at all. Dialysis required.

Signs you may have kidney disease

Here are the most evident signs that you may have kidney disease.

Pain in the lower back

When you move or stretch, you can have a localized discomfort close to your kidneys that does not go away or worsens. Kidney issues may result in discomfort in the lower back, which contains the kidneys on each side of the spine. Back discomfort may also result from an infection or kidney obstruction, which can harm the kidneys.

A decreased appetite

You could lose your appetite because of feeling full, being too ill or exhausted to eat, or because of a buildup of toxins brought on by decreased renal function.

To make urine, healthy kidneys filter blood. Urination problems, such as the desire to pee more frequently or noticing blood in your urine, can happen when the kidneys are not working correctly. Additionally, you may see frothy or bubbly pee, which might indicate that protein is entering your urine because of damaged kidneys.

Fatigue

You may have low energy or extreme fatigue due to a buildup of toxins in the blood because of impaired kidney function. Anemia, which results from having too few red blood cells, can make you feel exhausted or weak and may also be brought on by CKD.

Itching

If you have dry and itchy skin, you may have a mineral and nutritional imbalance in your blood because of renal illness. High amounts of phosphorus in the blood may induce itching.

Swelling in hands, legs, or feet

Edema, often known as swelling, can develop in your feet or other lower limbs when your kidneys are not eliminating too much salt and moisture from your body.

Difficulty in breathing

When your kidneys are not draining enough fluid, extra fluid might accumulate in your lungs, making you feel out of breath. Breathlessness may also be brought on by CKD-induced Anemia, a deficiency in red blood cells that deliver Oxygen.

Abnormal amounts of calcium, phosphorus, or vitamin D

Electrolyte imbalances brought on by impaired kidney function, such as low calcium levels or excessive phosphorus, can result in muscular cramps.

Abnormal urine test

Proteinuria, or high protein levels in the urine, is a symptom of renal disease. Protein escapes into your urine when the kidneys are not working correctly. Protein can re-enter circulation when the kidneys are healthy and filter out waste and moisture.

Elevated blood pressure

You may experience elevated blood pressure because of the extra fluid and salt buildup brought on by renal illness. In addition to harming renal blood vessels, high blood pressure can eventually aggravate kidney disease. [4] [5]

Can the Current Stage of Kidney Disease be Established Based on the presence of metabolic wastes like Creatinine and BUN

BUN blood urea nitrogen is between 70 to 20 mg/dl or 2.5 and 7.1 mmol/L. There is no definite value of BUN that would diagnose kidney failure. The test may be done with other tests to support the diagnosis of a kidney condition or measure how well your kidney disease medications are working. [6] Depending on your age, gender, medical history, and other factors, test results may differ. Depending on the lab utilized, your test results might change. They could not indicate an issue with you. Ask your healthcare practitioner to determine what your test finding signifies for you.

A average BUN level considered normal ranges from 7 to 20 milligrams per deciliter (mg/dL). This level may only help your doctor assess the health of your kidneys unless it is higher than 60 mg/dL. The ratio of BUN to creatinine in your blood is a more accurate gauge. BUN to creatinine ratios should typically range from 10:1

4
5   https://www.freseniuskidneycare.com/kidney-disease/ckd/symptoms
6   https://www.urmc.rochester.edu/encyclopedia/content.aspx?contenttypeid=167&contentid=urea_nitrogen_serum

to 20:1. If it is lower or greater than that, you could have a kidney condition or not be drinking enough water, respectively. [7]

Various techniques for measuring BUN and creatinine have emerged over time. Most of those are automated and produce clinically accurate and repeatable findings.

Urea nitrogen can be measured using one of two techniques. The diacetyl, or Fearon, reaction produces a yellow chromogen with urea, which may be measured via photometry. It has been adapted for auto analyzers and makes typically reliable findings. However, it still has low selectivity, as seen by illusory increases with sulfonylurea drugs and colorimetric interference from hemoglobin when using whole blood. [8]

What is the BUN test?

Urea nitrogen levels are one indicator of how well your kidneys are operating. The quantity of urea nitrogen in your blood is measured by a blood urea nitrogen (BUN) test. This straightforward test involves collecting blood from your body via a vein in your arm. Urea is a waste product produced by the liver that goes via the bloodstream to the kidneys and is filtered out. It is then excreted from your body via urine. Because this process is continuous, a tiny quantity of urea in your blood is typical. Too much urea indicates it is not adequately filtered and may suggest renal disease.

---

7   https://www.urmc.rochester.edu/encyclopedia/content.aspx?contenttypeid=167&contentid=urea_nitrogen_serum
8   https://www.ncbi.nlm.nih.gov/books/NBK305/

What is the purpose of a blood urea nitrogen (BUN) test?

A BUN test is a regular test ordered by your doctor as part of a comprehensive metabolic panel (CMP) or basic metabolic panel (BMP) during your visit (BMP). If you are admitted to the emergency department or during a routine hospital stay, it will be done.

If you have risk factors for renal disease, the BUN test may be administered as a precaution. Early kidney disease has no symptoms; however, the following variables might increase your risk: Kidney illness runs in the family.

- Hypertension Diabetes (high blood pressure)
- Cardiovascular disease Blood pressure is high.
- If your doctor believes you have kidney illness, they may conduct a BUN test.
- The symptoms that mandated a test are mentioned below:
- Frequent urination or insufficient urination
- Fatigue
- Urine that is colored or otherwise peculiar (bloody, foamy, coffee-colored)
- Swelling of the eyes, face, belly, arms, legs, or feet
- Vomiting or nausea [9]

The quantity of urea nitrogen in your blood is determined by a blood urea nitrogen (BUN) test. When your liver breaks down protein, urea nitrogen is produced as a waste product. Your blood carries it, your kidneys filter it out, and your urine excretes it from your body. Your liver may not properly break down proteins if it is not in good shape. Additionally, unhealthy kidneys may be unable to filter urea as well. Higher urea nitrogen levels may develop in your

---

9   https://my.clevelandclinic.org/health/diagnostics/17684-blood- urea-nitrogen-bun-test

body because of either of these issues. BUN plays an essential role in kidney diseases.

Does the treatment during the End Stage of Renal Disease depend on the dialysis machine's parameters like Time, Volume, and BFR to obtain the Blood Liters Processed for the Adequacy of the Dialysis?

The main factors determining the type of dialysis for people with chronic kidney disease are patient preferences about the treatment that best suits their lifestyle, availability of options within a service, and clinical contraindications.

When we talk about dialysis, two main types of dialysis are available, Hemodialysis and peritoneal dialysis. The factors that patients and caregivers may need to consider about peritoneal dialysis are the ability to carry out dialysis themselves; the support services they need to carry out dialysis; integration of dialysis with work, school, hobbies, and social and family activities; opportunities to maintain social contacts; possible modifications to their home; the distance and time traveling to the hospital; flexibility of daily treatment, diet, and medication regimens; and potential changes to body image and physical activities because of dialysis access points.[10]

Adequate dialysis is essential for reducing morbidity and mortality among patients requiring Hemodialysis. Kt/V is referred to as the used marker for dialysis adequacy. Kt/V is modifiable through different factors, such as dialyzer dialysis frequency, duration of dialysis, dialysate flow rate, and dialyzer blood flow rate (BFR).

---

10   https://pubmed.ncbi.nlm.nih.gov/22536622/

BFR is essential for achieving adequate Kt/V in 4th and end-stage chronic kidney failure. Increasing BFR while keeping the same surface, dialysate flow leads to a 23% increase in urea clearance. Hence, lower BFR causes inadequate dialysis outcomes.

The BFR, if kept below 250 ml during Hemodialysis, may increase mortality for chronic HD patients. Hence, monitoring the factors boosting the BFR is essential as they will help improve the results.

Which is the best nutritional supplement for CKD patients that contains lesser sugar?

Sugar intake, particularly in the form of fructose, has been linked to renal damage. Because their compositions are comparable, there is no evidence that sucrose is safer for the kidney than high fructose corn syrup (HFCS). So far, five epidemiologic studies have directly examined the link between sugar consumption (through sugar-sweetened drinks) and CKD. Although most research implies that sugar-sweetened beverage consumption increases the risk of CKD, only a few studies find statistically significant relationships.

How Much Water to Drink: An Integral Part in Kidney Health in Pediatric, Adulthood, And Geriatric of Healthy People and Dialysis Patients Regarding Ph Balance and Hydration?

Be "water wise" to protect the health of your kidneys. This involves consuming the appropriate Volume of water for you. The amount of water you require depends on your age, the environment where you live, how hard you exercise, and whether you are a dialysis patient, adult, or healthy person. Everyone is different. Thus, each person's daily water requirements will vary. It is a widespread misunderstanding that everyone should drink eight glasses of water daily.

The kidneys control the Volume and makeup of body fluids. Fundamental regulatory mechanisms involving the kidneys are described on this page for regulating volume, sodium and potassium concentrations, and pH of body fluids. The kidneys are the primary site of controlled water excretion, with the skin, lungs, and faces losing approximately a liter of water daily. Understanding how sodium and water control work together to protect the body from any potential changes in the Volume and osmolality of physiological fluids is crucial for you to understand. Dehydration, blood loss, salt consumption, and plain water consumption are some disorders. Water balance is established in the body by ensuring that the amount of water taken by food and drink (and produced by metabolism) balances the amount of water expelled. The behavioral processes that control consumption include salt and thirst desires.

The abrupt onset of acute renal failure and its frequent reversibility. Accidents, injuries, illnesses, infections, shock, and drug or poison consumption are a few causes. The kidneys stop making urine when they are injured. As poisons accumulate in the bloodstream, the patient becomes confused, unconscious, and bloated. Kidney function could improve with treatment, while chronic kidney failure occurs gradually and typically cannot be reversed. A diet, hydration restrictions, and temporary dialysis are prescribed to patients with acute renal failure until their kidneys have healed. Dialysis is typically necessary if the disease has advanced and the kidneys no longer function at 10% to 15% of normal levels. Even though dialysis carries out some of the activities of healthy kidneys, it does not treat kidney disease. The patient will typically require kidney transplantation or dialysis for the remainder of their life.

Acute kidney injury (AKI) within the first 48 hours following the occurrence, serum creatinine rises by 0.3%, blood urea nitrogen

(BUN) also increases, and glomerular filtration rate (GFR) rapidly falls within hours to days.

Are Condiments like Salt Resulting in HTN and Sugar in DM behind Acute/Chronic Kidney Failure?

High blood sugar resulting from diabetes leads to damaged blood vessels in the kidney. Each kidney consists of millions of tiny filters known as nephrons. Resultantly, nephrons are also affected and cease to function as they should. Also, diabetes may lead to high blood pressure (hypertension), along with diabetes mellitus are some of the significant risk factors for chronic kidney failure. These two factors account for 70% of end-stage kidney disease cases.

Condiments like salt (sodium) increase blood pressure, so a low-salt diet is recommended for all those suffering from hypertension. The recommended intake is a maximum of 2400 mg to 3000 mg. To make it easier to understand, any food with more than 400mg of sodium per serving will fall under the category of high sodium. Salt intake is associated with impaired kidney function among the general population, especially those with diabetes mellitus and hypertension. Salt intake is associated with developing chronic kidney disease and affects blood pressure. It also affects the eGFR, which means the estimated glomerular filtration rate. eFGR measures the effectiveness of the kidneys. It offers an estimated number, considering factors such as age, race, body type, etc.

Effects of medications containing salt compounds given to patients with low Bp, aside from NaCl saline bags?

Providing healthy blood pressure will ensure adequate oxygen supply to the brain tissue. Medications containing salt cause your blood volume to expand by ensuring fluid retention in the venous circulatory system, thereby not allowing the blood pressure to drop. This will ensure there are no episodes of syncope.

Tips to prevent kidney failure

Kidneys can be kept healthy by addressing the risk factors. By managing risk factors, all individuals can prevent the onset of chronic kidney disease and other associated complications. According to the CDC, the following tips help contain the threat of CKD.

- Losing weight if you are obese
- Being physically active as it helps control blood sugar levels
- Quit smoking
- Getting checked regularly to ensure your kidney is healthy
- Take medications as prescribed and directed by the doctor
- Maintaining blood pressure below 140/90
- Those who have diabetes need to stay in the recommended blood sugar range
- Do not exceed the target cholesterol range
- Consume foods containing less salt
- Consuming a diet of fruits and vegetables

How to manage CKD

If you are already suffering from CKD, then you need to implement the following changes

- Healthy eating by conforming to a renal diet as proposed by a dietician
- Taking proper medications

- Avoiding medications and kidney infections that may cause harm to the kidneys. Medications that need to be avoided include over-the-counter pain medications, such as ibuprofen and naproxen, and certain antibiotics
- Dyes used for making organs or blood vessels visible on X-rays and other imaging tests

Is Stem Cell Therapy for Kidney Failure an excellent alternative to a Kidney Transplant?

Stem cell therapy can benefit patients suffering from moderate to late/terminal stage renal failure by removing the need for dialysis or reducing the frequency of dialysis. Stem cell treatment can repair kidney damage and prevent additional harm to renal function in patients with early-stage renal failure or kidney disease. Our functional regenerative medical therapies employing improved renal stem cells allow patients the certainty that their kidneys will not deteriorate or spread to cause other concerns such as heart disease (heart attacks), pancreatic failure (diabetic nephropathy), and other complications. [11]Although it is challenging to regenerate the kidney in vitro completely, recent developments in the field of S.C.s have made it possible to create organoids in vitro. When creating new kidney tissues for transplantation, induced pluripotent stem cells are the most significant source because they can potentially come from patients and be utilized as a renal replacement therapy without immunosuppression. Based on research when creating fresh kidney tissues for transplantation, induced pluripotent stem cells are the ideal source because they can potentially come from patients and be utilized as a renal replacement therapy without immunosuppression. [12]

---

11 https://stemcellthailand.org/therapies/renal-failure-kidney-disease/
12 https://www.healthcentral.com/article/collagen-supplements-and-kidneys

CHAPTER TWO:
PARTICIPATING IN THE DIALYSIS

Albumin as an Indicator of Diseases Apart from Nutritional Deficiency in Adults

Albumin refers to a protein found in the blood plasma of humans. An albumin test helps detect the liver and kidneys' functioning levels. If low albumin levels are found in the test, it could result from kidney disease. However, other reasons, such as liver disease, infections, or inflammation, are also possible. Low albumin levels are mainly detected due to severe diarrhea or dehydration.

If low levels of albumin are detected in the body, then the doctor will try to find the exact reason behind the cause. This is because albumin levels also indicate underlying nutritional deficits, such as low protein in the patient's diet.

To detect a cause other than nutritional defects, a patient may be required to undergo blood tests or urine tests in addition to the albumin blood test. Low albumin levels possibly point out to kidney disease if the following symptoms are also present:

- Appetite loss
- Fatigue
- Trouble concentrating
- Frequent need to urinate
- Dry or itchy skin

- Muscle cramps
- Weakness
- Vomiting or nausea
- Swelling in the face, ankle, or feet
- Urine changes

Ferritin and kidneys

Ferritin helps protect a kidney after the effects of a damaging injury by controlling body's iron levels. Ferritin is a blood protein containing iron, and a ferritin test is carried out to measure the amount of Ferritin present in your blood. With this test, your healthcare specialist can determine the amount of iron your body stores. If the blood ferritin level is lower than the normal range, you have an iron deficiency because your body's iron stores are low. However, Ferritin also has a link with the kidneys. High levels of Ferritin in your body could indicate CKD with glomerular disease and proteinuria.

Is Ferritin an inflammatory marker?

Though a ferritin test allows a doctor to discern the quantity of iron in your body, Ferritin is still a marker of inflammation. Instead of just being a marker of iron status in people who are overweight, ferritin levels are essential in determining subclinical inflammation.

Ferritin levels are elevated in inflammation. These increased Ferritin levels indicate the important host defense mechanism during infection. This mechanism is essential for depriving bacterial growth of iron. It also protects immune cell function. Since it is protective, it limits free radical production.

It is also important to note that high or low levels of Ferritin may not necessarily indicate a medical condition that requires treatment. Around 1 in 20 healthy people will give results beyond Ferritin's normal range.

Managing Vegan Protein diet for Kidneys in CKD and dialysis patients

If the patient already has CSK, plant-based foods help slow down the progression of not just CSK but Type 2 diabetes, high blood pressure, and heart disease. Including plant-based proteins in your diet, such as vegetables and grains, can contribute to your kidney health. Replacing red meat with vegetable products helps prevent chronic kidney disease.

Studies also indicate that a diet rich in whole grains, fruits, vegetables, and nuts helps keep the kidney healthy. However, suggesting that a plant-based diet does not imply quitting all animal protein sources is also important. Having CSK or being put on dialysis does not require a person on a vegetarian diet to start consuming animal protein. If you are on dialysis, you need a kidney diet with a proper meal plan to help in both dialysis processes and fulfilling your nutritional needs. You must monitor your calorie intake to avoid a deficit in your needed calories. Your diet will need vegetarian protein sources, possibly calorie supplements when required. Phosphate binders will need to be increased when taking meals and snacks. It is essential that while on dialysis, you need a lower potassium dialysate so that the potassium levels can be kept in control. The diet will also need to be adjusted for acceptable levels of urea clearance.

Plant-based foods help slow the decline of GFR, glomerular filtration rate, and kidney blood flow. It also helps reduce kidney cyst growth and improves the lipid profile of the blood, known as blood fat.

Though patients in the initial stages of kidney disease are advised to limit the intake of proteins, dialysis patients would need more protein. This is because more protein loss occurs during dialysis. For vegetarians on dialysis, ensuring enough protein intake while controlling potassium and phosphorus is complex and may require a protein supplement.

Collagen-based protein in Dialysis and Kidney Transplant patients

Your body naturally produces collagen, a protein that keeps your connective tissues, such as your muscles, tendons, ligaments, and cartilage, solid and flexible. The most prevalent protein in the human body is collagen.

However, as you age, your body produces less collagen naturally. According to a study, collagen synthesis begins to halt in your 20s and declines at a rate of 1% every year after that. A wide range of additional lifestyle factors, such as excessive alcohol consumption, insufficient sleep, inactivity, and U.V. exposure, can significantly affect output.

While collagen supplements could be advantageous, some people may find them risky. Knowing how the body metabolizes collagen is necessary to comprehend the potential connection between collagen supplements and renal problems such as kidney stones.

Dr. David P. Selzer, a nephrologist at NYU Langone Medical Associates in West Palm Beach, FL, notes that supplements containing collagen protein include the amino acid hydroxyproline, which the body metabolizes into oxalate. The human body is unable to decompose the simple chemical molecule oxalate further.

Why is the CVC prone to bacterial/fungi infection?

Compared to other medical devices, central venous catheters (CVCs) have the highest risk of device-related infections and significantly contribute to morbidity and mortality. Bloodstream infections linked to central venous catheters are a significant source of hospital-acquired infections linked to morbidity, death, and expense. The severity of the effects depends on the linked organisms, underlying pre-morbid states, timeliness, and suitability of the given treatment or intervention. The prevalence of indwelling medical devices, antineoplastic/immunosuppressive medications, central venous catheters (CVC), and other indwelling devices contributes to an increase in the incidence of opportunistic infections by filamentous fungus. This case involves a 13-year-old kid receiving therapy for acute lymphoblastic leukemia. Due to an intermittent fever with no recognized cause, the kid was readmitted to the pediatric ward. The cultures' results were compared through the CVC or peripheral venous sites.

Gram-negative organisms are responsible for 20–30% of CRBSI infections. Between 40% and 80% of CRBSIs are brought on by gram-positive bacteria. Coagulase-negative, the most prevalent microorganisms are Staphylococci, Staphylococcus aureus, and Enterococcus. Staphylococci resistant to methicillin are common.

What are the factors that inoculate these organisms?

Thousands of people die each year from central line-associated bloodstream infections (CLABSIs), which contribute billions of dollars to the cost of healthcare in the United States despite being preventable. To aid in eradicating CLABSIs, the CDC offers recommendations and resources to the medical community.

Prevention through handwashing

Since CVCs cause almost 90% of infections related to caterers, its essential to practice proper hygienic measures. CVCs are also integral to hemodynamic monitoring. Hand hygiene is recognized as the most effective and cost-effective way of reducing infection. Hand hygiene is essential for reducing infection rates. According to the World Health Organization, there are "Five Moments for Hand Hygiene." Hand hygiene must be followed, with hands washed with alcohol-based sanitizer on five accounts. These are before the patient is touched and cleaning is performed. The hands must be rewashed after the patient is exposed to the body fluid. Hands must be washed after touching the patient and after you have come in contact with the patient's surroundings.

CVCs infection rates in the U.S.

A 46% decrease in central line-associated bloodstream infections (CLABSI) was witnessed in hospitals across the U.S. during 2008-2013. However, around 30,100 CLABSIs occur in ICUs and other wards of hospitals each year.

CLABSI prevention measures through prevention programs help reduce the risk of infections, and nursing education should continue to benefit from a further reduction in CLABSI.

PARTICIPATING IN THE DIALYSIS 31

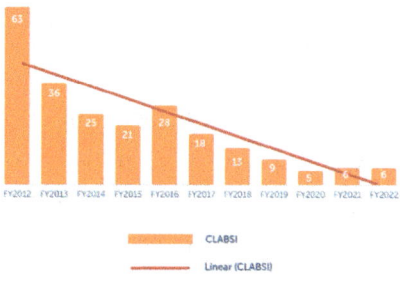

Use of Povidone-Iodine and Alcohol Prep to Kill Bacteria, Fungi, and Mycobacteria and Viruses

In the past six decades, povidone-iodine (PVP-I) formulations have helped minimize the impact and spread of infectious diseases. These diseases include ones with potent antiviral, antibacterial, and antifungal effects.

When alcohol is used for disinfection, many bacteria will remain active. In contrast, povidone iodine offers a broad range of protection against bacteria, fungi, and viruses. It has demonstrated the rapid and substantive disinfecting effect in CVCs.

Cooling Dialysate Solution at room temperature to avoid moisture and the resulting growth of fungi and microorganisms

There needs to be temperature control in dialysis to prevent heat accumulation, which would increase the body temperature during Hemodialysis. Cooling dialysate has been utilized to ensure peripheral vasoconstriction on dialysis. It helps reduce the incidence of intradialytic hypotension.

Body temperature cooling is essential to stabilize BP and reduce intradialytic events, which may require staff intervention. It helps avoid compromising the efficacy of treatment and ensures high-efficiency dialysis. This way, the moisture can be controlled. The growth of fungi and microorganisms can also be controlled by controlling moisture. The standard temperature is 37°C (98.6°F), the average dialysate temperature for long-term hemodialysis patients.

Preventing the growth of fungi in case the GT supplement contains a high amount of sugar

Different factors render people prone to Candida infections. These include diabetes and a weak immune system. A low-sugar diet is also essential to controlling yeast infection. If the consumed GT supplements have much sugar, it will lead to the growth of fungi. Increased sugar intake promotes the growth of fungi.

Diflucan (fluconazole), an oral medication, is taken in one dose: other available OTC (over-the-counter medicines) or medications, such as butoconazole (Gynazole). In case of severe infection and a high sugar intake, a longer prescription course would be required, such as GT supplements.

Importance of maintaining the Baseline of the BP

Baseline blood pressure (BP) is a marker of response to antihypertensive therapy. It is used to calculate the patient's ability to reach BP goals. Since blood pressure increases in end-stage renal diseases and those on dialysis resulting in a high incidence of cardiovascular diseases, it is vital to keep the blood pressure regular around the baseline BP to avoid reduced lifespan of hemodialysis patients.

Hypertension is a common condition among chronic kidney disease patients. In most cases, it remains poorly controlled in hemodialysis patients. Sodium and volume excess are the two most important factors that cause hypertension in dialysis patients. Hence, non-pharmacologic strategies are required to control the BP and reach the BP baseline. These include the individualized dialysate sodium prescription. Another option available is the gradual dry-weight reduction. To ensure a patient lives longer on Hemodialysis, it is important to maintain the BP baseline.

Time management in Hemodialysis

Hemodialysis can be performed at home or in-center. A nurse or a technician carries out in-center hemodialysis, typically performed thrice weekly, with each session lasting three to four hours or more. However, the time needs to be planned before as it is usually pre-scheduled,

Hemodialysis can also be carried out at home, where you can fit the treatment into your schedule.

At home, you have many options. You may opt for conventional home dialysis, which requires you to undergo sessions of three to four hours or longer three times every week. There is also the short daily home hemodialysis, where sessions are performed five to seven times every week, with each treatment lasting two hours. The third option is that nocturnal home hemodialysis is performed at night while you sleep. It lasts six to eight hours and needs to be done six nights a week, every second night, depending on what the doctor prescribes for you.

When it comes to short daily Hemodialysis, there are many added benefits. It requires the patient to take fewer medications to control blood pressure and Anemia and keep phosphorus under control. It also results in an improvement in neuropathy and embanking nerve damage and also reduces restless leg syndrome. Patients typically have more energy for daily tasks and can sleep better. This leads to improvement in life quality and allows patients to live longer. It also results in fewer and shorter stays at the hospital.

Studies have also indicated that fewer hours of delivered dialysis led to a higher systolic Blood pressure, and four hours of dialysis per session led to a reduction in systolic blood pressure with fewer dialysis sessions.

Fungal growth occurs optimally at room temperatures, around 25 c. In higher temperatures, lower change occurs. Fungal contamination in the dialysate solution poses a severe risk to those requiring dialysis treatment. The risk is higher because of the debilitated immune system of such patients. Hemodialysis, the primary treatment for such patients, is carried out thrice a week, mostly in sessions of around 3–4 hours. The period depends on the patient's clinical condition. The problem is that during these sessions, water is utilized to produces dialysate. Water is also used in the reuse of dialyzers. A patient will be exposed to approximately 400 liters of water weekly during the hemodialysis sessions. Hence, ensuring good water quality is essential for reducing the risks exposed to the patient's health.

Hypotension in dialysis patients: Why does it occur and how to treat it

Hypotension during dialysis or dialysis hypotension occurs because of inadequate cardiovascular response to the reduction in blood volume during the dialysis process. The decrease in blood volume is due removing a large volume of water within a short span. Hypotension during dialysis is linked directly to the reduction in blood volume. It can also be said that it is connected to decreased cardiovascular activation. Cardiovascular activation occurs in response to decreased cardiac filling. The decreased cardiovascular activation is either linked to the patient or dialysis-related factors.

During Hemodialysis, hypotension is common. To treat this issue, the patient needs intravenous fluid replacement. This way, the patients can be made to leave the dialysis unit safely.

Ensuring a stable Fluid Balance through Dry Weight (weight equal to Volume)

To ensure dialysis is adequately conducted, Fluid Volume and hemodynamic management are essential for the health of hemodialysis patients. Salt and water homeostasis management is necessary and is undertaken by the 'dry weight' approach.

This clinical approach has been demonstrated to offer benefits for cardiovascular outcomes. The effect of cardiovascular filling has already been discussed in the above section on hypotension in dialysis patients.

It is important to note that a more precise approach must be adopted to improve cardiovascular outcomes in high-risk populations. For this purpose, fluid status assessment and monitoring must rely on four essential components. These are:

- Clinical assessment
- Non-invasive instrumental tools, such as blood volume monitoring
- Cardiac biomarkers
- Algorithm and sodium modeling for estimating the mass transfer

For optimal management of fluid and sodium imbalance, the salt and fluid removal by dialysis must be adjusted with ultrafiltration and dialysate sodium. Also, the salt intake and fluid gain during the dialysis session must be restricted.

The handling of sodium and water must be ensured in a precise and personalized way. For this purpose, modern technology can be utilized, such as biosensors, feedback control tools, and sophisticated analytics.

For managing the health of patients requiring dialysis, it must be noted that the 'dry weight' policy is needed when you view the case from a clinical perspective. However, the dry weight policy is insufficient to ensure a full cardioprotective effect when you view it from a pathophysiologic standpoint. For this reason, a more balanced and precise approach must be adopted to improve cardiovascular outcomes. Healthcare workers must move towards a broader approach to meet this need. Hence, comprehensive hemodynamic management of such patients must be provided instead of focusing only on the fluid management of dialysis patients. When examining an individual's euvolemic condition, weight, and fluid quantities are inextricably linked, especially in the context of dialysis patients. Euvolemia is where the body's fluid volume is suitable and balanced.

Dialysis patients must maintain euvolemia since fluid excess and dehydration may harm their health. The quantity of fluid consumption permitted is calculated case-by-case, considering various criteria. These considerations include the patient's general health, residual renal function, urine output, dietary limitations, and concomitant medical disorders. This helps avoid excess fluid, which may cause edema, shortness of breath, elevated blood pressure, and cardiovascular strain.

The ultrafiltration rate determines the fluid is removed from the patient's circulation during dialysis. By closely monitoring these indicators, healthcare practitioners may alter the ultrafiltration rate to remove the proper quantity of fluid, assisting the patient in achieving and maintaining euvolemic status.

Weight is a practical and readily quantifiable sign of fluid status changes. Healthcare practitioners weigh patients before and after dialysis treatments to assess the efficacy of fluid removal and overall fluid balance. Sudden weight increases between dialysis sessions may suggest excessive fluid retention, prompting changes to the patient's fluid restriction and ultrafiltration rate during the following dialysis sessions.

Fluid management in dialysis patients needs a specific, multifaceted strategy. To identify the patient's fluid status, healthcare personnel thoroughly examine their clinical symptoms, blood pressure, and laboratory findings. By considering these aspects, healthcare practitioners may make educated judgments about fluid intake limitations and fluid removal during dialysis sessions. Dialysis patients must actively engage in their fluid management. Patients and their healthcare teams must communicate and collaborate regularly to optimize fluid management techniques, reduce consequences of fluid imbalances, and improve the patient's overall quality of life.

In conclusion, weight and fluid volumes are critical in determining dialysis patients' euvolemic states. Fluid intake limitation and dialysis fluid removal are two primary strategies for maintaining fluid balance. Healthcare practitioners may adjust fluid management techniques to each patient's requirements by regularly monitoring weight and other pertinent data, guaranteeing euvolemia and lowering the risk of problems associated with fluid imbalances.

CHAPTER THREE:
ROOT CAUSES OF THE DIALYSIS PROBLEMS

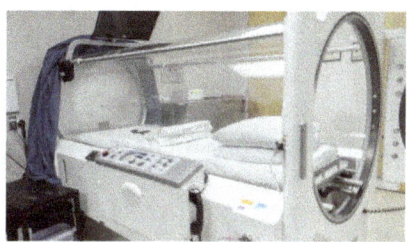

What is Hyperbaric Oxygen Therapy, and why it needs to be a part of the Dialysis Regimen to treat severe Anemia

A healthcare provider may recommend hyperbaric oxygen therapy (HBOT) to a patient for different conditions, such as brain abscesses and severe Anemia. This therapy may also be suggested to patients with air bubbles in their blood vessels, a condition known as arterial gas embolism.

Hyperbaric oxygen therapy is vital in treating kidney patients who suffer from Anemia and require dialysis. Including this therapy as part of the dialysis regimen makes the overall treatment plan more effective if the patient also has severe Anemia. This therapy has the potential to improve renal Hypoxia. It increases the partial pressure of dissolved (non-hemoglobin-bound) oxygen. This effect is observed without the demand for Oxygen being affected. This therapy is helpful as it recruits tissue and peripheral progenitors and ensures the optimal environment crucial for their proliferation and tissue repair.

Who should avoid Hyperbaric oxygen therapy?

However, Hyperbaric oxygen therapy does not suit everyone. This therapy must be avoided by those suffering from certain lung conditions or diseases. This is because offering therapy to such patients will increase the risk of a collapsed lung.

Anemia and Hyperbaric oxygen therapy

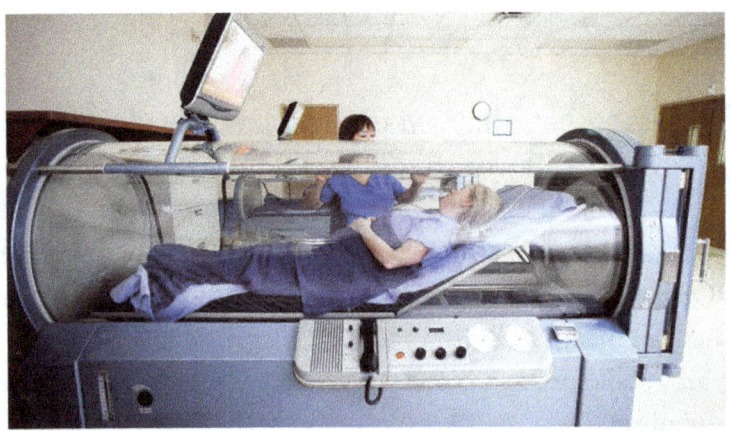

As mentioned above, Hyperbaric oxygen therapy is an integral part of the overall treatment plan for kidney patients who suffer from severe Anemia and need dialysis. Anemia is a condition in which the patient suffers from a lack of blood. In this condition, there is precisely a lack of red blood cells. Since there is a deficiency of red blood cells and hemoglobin, it means that the blood's oxygen-carrying capacity is severely affected. This causes severe symptoms, such as shock, pallor, fatigue, and weakness.

There are different causes of Anemia. These include excessive blood loss, which may result from internal bleeding or trauma. Another likely cause is the abnormal production of red blood cells in the bone marrow. The condition can also be caused by a disease's destruction of red blood cells.

Hyperbaric Oxygen Therapy helps push Oxygen to the vital organs of the body. This way, it addresses the problem of Anemia which is a life-threatening condition.

Treatment of gangrene

Hyperbaric oxygen therapy also helps alleviate conditions like gangrene. It speeds up the healing of carbon monoxide poisoning, wounds, and gangrene that are not healing. It also helps treat infections by providing Oxygen to tissues facing oxygen starvation.

There are different treatments for gangrene. These include oxygen therapy, antibiotics, and surgery. The purpose is to restore blood flow and eliminate dead tissue. However, it is important to identify gangrene in the initial stages as it improves the prospect of recovery.

Treatment of infections

Oxygen therapy helps treat different infections. It is also suitable for treating chronic infections. Examples include necrotizing fasciitis and osteomyelitis. Other conditions that can be treated include infective endocarditis and soft tissue infections.

Treatment of brain injury

HBOT also offers an effective treatment plan for brain injury. It can potentially improve chronic traumatic brain injury (TBI) symptoms permanently. It is worth noting that TBI happens to be one of the leading causes of death and injury in the U.S.

Supplementing Anemia medications (Mircera, Aranesp, and ESA) that have serious side effects in patients requiring dialysis

Iron is an essential mineral the body uses for growth and development that carries oxygen from the lungs to other body parts. In addition to this, iron helps in the manufacture of a protein known as myoglobin, which provides the muscles with oxygen. The iron mineral plays numerous vital functions in the body, such as providing general energy, strengthening the immune system, helping in gastrointestinal processes, and regulating body temperature. The benefits associated with iron are often noticed once an individual needs to get enough of the mineral, and its deficiency can lead to heart palpitations, fatigue, breathlessness, and pale skin. Moreover, iron improves cognition by restoring optimal bodily functions, thus increasing cognitive performance, focus, and memory.

The daily iron needs of women increase at the onset of adolescence because they lose blood each month with the start of menstruation. Women of all ages require more iron than men to maintain healthy iron levels. Iron also plays a crucial role in health and hair growth; therefore, adequate levels of the mineral help prevent hair loss in women. Additionally, pregnant women need a high amount of iron because the deficiency of this mineral increases the risk of having a preterm delivery or delivering a child with low birth weight. Women know if their bodies need energy when they experience fatigue, low energy, and heavy menstrual cycles that may indicate low iron.

Too much or too little iron affects the body as it could lead to blood pressure anomalies. Iron supplements with dietary sources do not prove any effect of supplementation on blood pressure. However, very high doses of iron, especially among children, can lead to low blood pressure and eventually death. Besides, nutritional iron supplements among children with low birth weight prevent the prevalence of hypertension during childhood years and later in adulthood. Supplements also assist in regulating iron levels in the body, and this helps to prevent blood pressure that affects the lungs and stabilizes red cells concentration in the blood.

Water and fiber should be balanced for dialysis patients to prevent side effects such as stomach pain and constipation when taking iron supplements and helps in the reduction of serum uremic toxins. Furthermore, dialysis patients should be encouraged to increase their fiber intake by eating pulses and lentils, wholegrain foods, and fruits and vegetables. Water and fiber can also be balanced by limiting the amount of salt in the diet. The body holds on to water due to salt; limiting salt helps control thirst. Moreover, the balance between fiber and water can be achieved by dividing water and fiber intake into manageable parts, such as taking several ounces of fluid and fiber portions at different intervals.

ESAs or erythropoiesis-stimulating agents increase the production of red blood cells by stimulating the bone marrow. These medications are used in treating Anemia resulting from chronic kidney failure and also due to some anticancer drugs. These medications are also helpful in reducing the blood transfusions required before or after major surgeries.

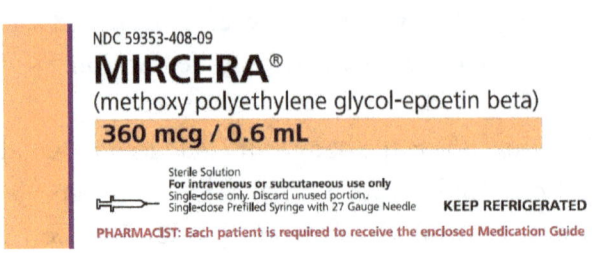
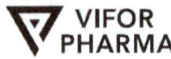

Mircera is an ESA used to treat Anemia stemming from chronic kidney disease in adults requiring or not requiring dialysis. However, it has many unpleasant side effects, such as headaches, diarrhea, body aches, and vomiting.

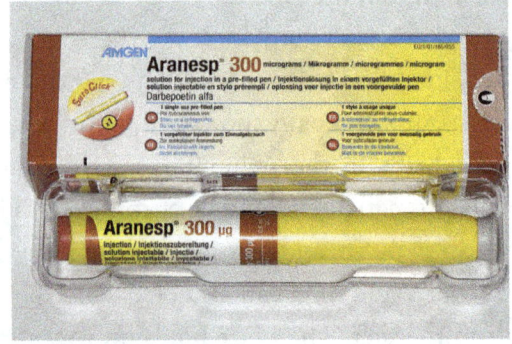

Aranesp is another medication used to treat Anemia. It, too, has many unpleasant side effects, such as cough and shortness of breath, and it causes low BP during dialysis.

Hyperbaric oxygen therapy is helpful as it can supplement these medicines with significant side effects.

Relationship between UTIs and diabetes

UTIs are urinary tract infections. These are infections caused by bacteria from the skin or rectum entering the urethra. These infections affect different parts of the urinary tract. However, the most common infection is bladder infection (cystitis). This causes infection in the urinary tract. Another type of UTI is known as pyelonephritis or Kidney infection.

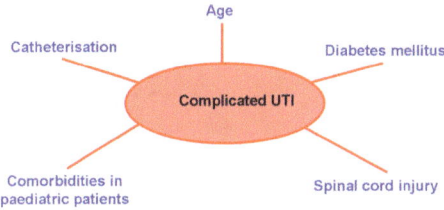

Diabetes has a close relation with urological health issues. People who have diabetes are vulnerable to contracting urinary tract infections. People with diabetes are also susceptible to bladder issues and sexual dysfunction. Diabetes is a debilitating condition that can worsen urologic conditions. This is because it affects the blood flow, besides hampering the sensory function of the body.

Psoriasis is an antibiotic found naturally that shields the body against the threat of UTIs. UTIs happen to be more common in people with diabetes. Diabetes causes high blood glucose levels, leading to a lack of psoriasis.

Increasing water intake to flush out bacteria in kidney dialysis patients

Drinking plenty of water and staying hydrated is necessary for kidney patients as it allows the body to remove bacteria and toxins naturally from the body. This way, drinking plenty of water can prevent illness.

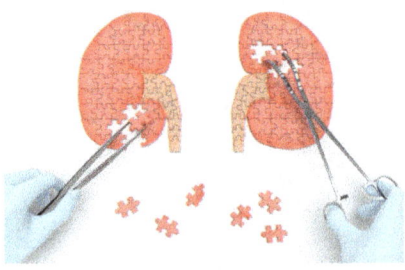

Drinking plenty of water during and after the infection helps flush out the system and prevents future infections. It also helps flush out bacteria that may otherwise reach the bladder and cause infection.

Filtration of hemodialysis fluids is also essential. This is because it effectively eliminates bacteria and prevents endotoxin contamination utilizing an oxidant, especially chlorine or peracetic acid, is the most suitable method to remove bacteria and endotoxins in dialysis. Other effective methods include the use of ozone and heat sanitization. Both these methods are FDA-approved for dialysis applications.

Since people with diabetes are more vulnerable to contracting urinary tract infections or suffer from bladder issues and sexual dysfunction, it is essential to exercise caution. Diabetes is a severe condition that worsens urologic conditions. This is because diabetes affects the body's blood flow and sensory function. UTIs are not only prevalent among those who have diabetes but are also more severe in such cases and can cause severe kidney problems. These include renal abscesses and emphysematous cystitis. It may also cause other complications, such as renal papillary necrosis.

Impact of Diabetes on the Body's immune system

For those who have type 1 diabetes, their pancreas may stop producing insulin. Insulin is required to regulate blood glucose levels. For people who have type 2 diabetes, their cells end up being less sensitive to insulin. In both these conditions, there is a high probability of excessive glucose levels accumulating in the blood. This, in turn, impacts the effectiveness of the immune system negatively. As mentioned earlier, high glucose levels due to diabetes lead to reduced levels of natural antibiotics found naturally in the human body, known as antimicrobial peptide psoriasis. This antibiotic serves as a shield against infection.

Urinary tract infections pose a more significant problem in patients with type 2 diabetes mellitus. Caused mainly by resistant pathogens, immune system impairments, and poor metabolic control increase the risk of UTIs in diabetic patients.

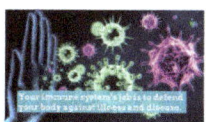

Dangers for chronic stable dialysis patients on account of infections like Staphylococcus Aureus

Dialysis patients are exposed to many dangers. As such, the risk of exposure to Staphylococcus aureus is also present among patients who undergo dialysis in various settings, such as dialysis centers, hospitals, or even rest homes. The underlying issue is that the vascular access needed during Hemodialysis becomes a potential entry site for S. aureus. This risk is magnified when healthcare givers use a central venous catheter (CVC). This increases the risk of contracting Sepsis when you compare it to arteriovenous (A.V.) fistula.

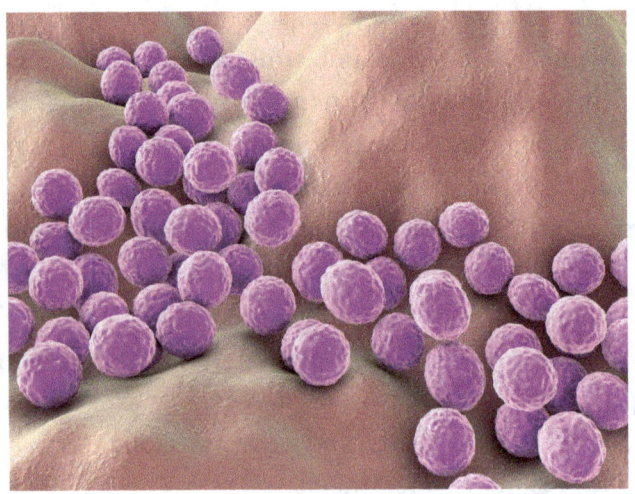

Activating the immune system's response

Staphylococcus aureus infects the bloodstream. For patients on Hemodialysis, this infection can have serious repercussions. The Human body's immune system responds against S. aureus by activating innate and adaptive immune systems. The innate immune response is the human body's first line of action to fight against the infection. This activation occurs more rapidly, opening the way to different pathways involved in detecting the nonspecific markers of microbial infection.

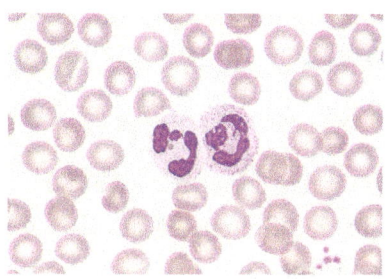

Neutrophils are white cells recognized as chemotaxis. These are the human body's second line of nonspecific defense. As part of the human immune system, they play an essential role in acute reactions and are a vital source of S. aureus.

It may surprise you, but 1 in 5 humans have been persistently colonized with Staphylococcus aureus bacteria. This is one of the leading causes behind the emergence of skin infections. It is also one of the main reasons for hospital-acquired infections, such as the antibiotic-resistant strain MRSA.

S. epidermidis is one of the members of the coagulase-negative Staphylococci. It is recognized as a critical commensal organism in the human skin. It is also found on the mucous membranes. Research has concluded that it helps human health because of its ability to fight harmful microorganisms. However, it also has some benefits for the human body.

The issue with patients who need to be kept on dialysis is that they often have weaker immune systems. This makes it difficult for such patients to fight off infections. Despite this setback, kidney patients cannot afford to forego their regularly scheduled dialysis treatments. This makes it mandatory that the precautions recommended by healthcare professionals be adhered to completely.

The importance of Mucus or phlegm having different mechanisms for the Human body

Medically, Mucus may have one name, but in our daily conversation, it is referred to by different names. It could be the snot, the sticky goo coming out the nose when a person has a cold. It could be phlegm, the gunk with the irritable side effect of clogging your lungs, resulting in a cough.

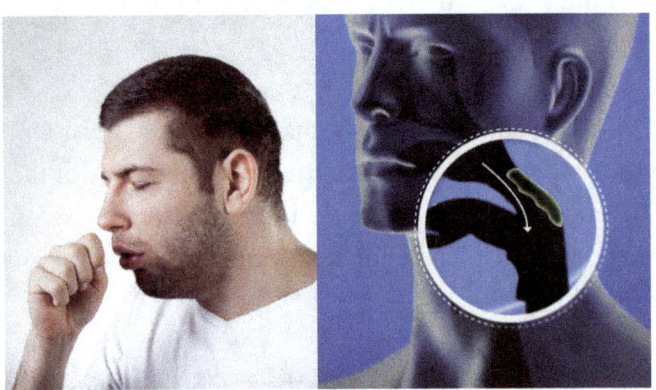

The Mucus plays a vital role in the Human body. Found in the respiratory tract, it warms the inhaled air and moistens it. It also ensures that the mucus membrane cells and hairs remain lubricated. It acts as a barrier that also defends the Human body. It has a layer that traps pathogens, including possible infectious microorganisms and other irritant particles. By doing so, it prevents them from entering the lungs.

The mucous membranes produce phlegm. Running from the nose to the lungs, it has an important function. The Mucus helps trap the viruses, allergens, and dust that the human body breathes in whenever it inhales air. All of these are blown out of the system during exhalation. However, in some cases, the body may produce a lot of Mucus. This leads to the need to cough frequently to clear the throat.

Does the color of the phlegm signify infection?

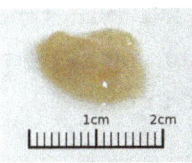

The color change depends on the severity and duration of the sickness. If the color of the phlegm is yellow or green, it may indicate that the human body is currently fighting infection and the color has come from the white blood cells. The phlegm usually reveals a yellow color which then turns green later.

Ways to treat excess mucus and phlegm buildup

Heating and drying out the passageways help overcome this problem. Such procedures are usually adopted in nursing homes. There is also the option of addressing the limited fluid intake required from dialysis patients.

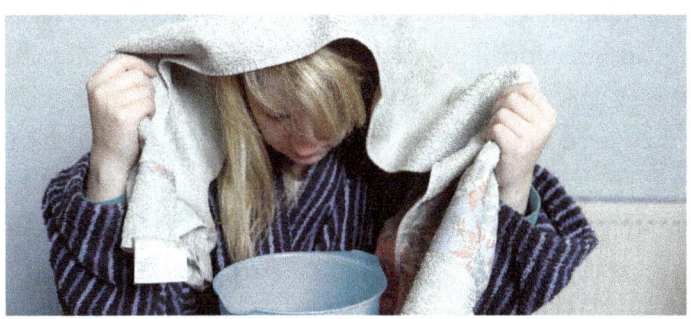

It is essential to keep the body hydrated to ensure the Mucus remains thin. If an individual falls sick, increasing fluid intake does the needful by thinning the Mucus and draining the sinuses.

An easy solution to this condition is spending time in a steam-filled bathroom. This will ensure that the Mucus in the nose and throat is loosened and cleared. Splashing hot water on the face also offers relief from sinus pressure.

Relief can also be obtained from a warm and wet washcloth. Heat plays a critical part in relieving pain and pressure. It alleviates the pounding sinus headache. Carrying out inhaling with a damp cloth is another effective way of moisturizing the nose and throat.

Boosting the immune support of Dialysis Patients through medicinal and nutritional supplements

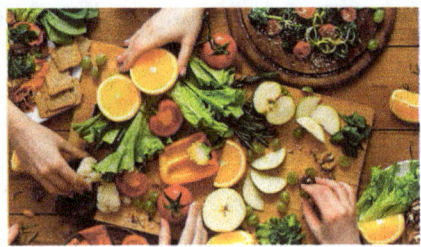

Patients requiring dialysis treatment are at an increased risk of contracting an infection. The risk of suffering invasion from pathogens is also high. Hemodialysis patients are vulnerable to infection because they need to undergo hemodialysis frequently, which involves using catheters. At times, it may also involve the insertion of needles. Healthcare professionals utilize these to access the bloodstream.

Supplements dialysis patients need to take

Kidney patients require a high intake of some water-soluble vitamins. This is why some particular renal vitamins need to be consumed by kidney patients. This is necessary for providing extra water-soluble vitamins to the body. Renal vitamins consist of vitamins such as B1, B2, B6, B12, niacin, folic acid, biotin, a small dose of vitamin C, and pantothenic acid.

Ways for dialysis patients to improve immunity

Different nutritional sources boost the immune system, and as such, they are essential for Kidney health. Leafy greens are an important source, especially the ones that include food sources like spinach and kale. Another vital source is Omega-3 fatty acids. These are critical fats involved in supporting cell functioning.

Other sources are known as the powerhouse of vitamins, such as blueberries and strawberries. Patients suffering from chronic kidney disease and requiring dialysis must abstain from consuming herbal remedies and over-the-counter supplements. This is because such sources may cause undesirable interactions when prescription medicines are also being taken.

Role of Seaweeds/Algae in aiding the Immune system of Dialysis Patients to fight off pathogens

Seaweeds and microalgae consist of pharmacologically active compounds. The phlorotannins, peptides, terpenes, fatty acids, and polysaccharides help fight against bacterial invasion.

Seaweed is involved in the production of metabolites that help in the fight against various environmental stressors. These compounds demonstrate different properties beneficial to the human body, such as antiviral, antibacterial, antiprotozoal, and antifungal properties.

Tips on boosting the immune systems of dialysis patients

Consume a diet containing more vitamin A. This is a kidney-friendly food source. Examples include carrots, broccoli, eggs, and red bell peppers. An intake of vitamin C is also recommended. Sources include melons, berries, bell peppers, and citrus fruits. Vitamin E is essential in seeds, nuts, cereals, and peanut butter.

Many options are also available for keeping your diet full of protein. These include beef, chicken, beans, eggs, lamb, fish, turkey, veal, and lentils. However, opting for natural, fresh meat is highly recommended, though frozen or canned meat is also a good option.

Sepsis in brief: Symptoms, entry points, potential to cause damage, and need to control

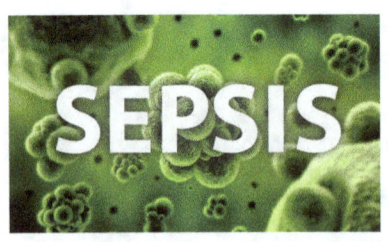

Sepsis refers to the body's extreme response in reaction to an infection. Sepsis occurs when an already present infection triggers a chain reaction all over the body. Most infections cause Sepsis to start in organs like the lungs, skin, or urinary tract. It is a severe issue that is life-threatening and requires urgent medical attention.

Symptoms

Here are some of the symptoms of Sepsis:

- Breathlessness
- Loss of consciousness
- A high or low body temperature
- Confusion or disorientation
- Slurred speech.
- Cold and pale skin.
- Heavy heartbeat.
- Fast breathing

Sepsis may also lead to tissue damage, organ failure, and death. Professionals call for implementing safety protocols to keep the infection in check. These include assessing the sites of the body accessed during Hemodialysis via X-rays.

Response of the immune system to Sepsis and inflammation

The Human body's immune system restricts an infection to one place, known as localized infection. This is ensured by the white blood cells produced by the body. White blood cells respond to an infection by traveling to the site to eliminate the germs responsible for the infection. This process allows the body to fight infection and prevent its spread. This process leads to tissue swelling, referred to as inflammation.

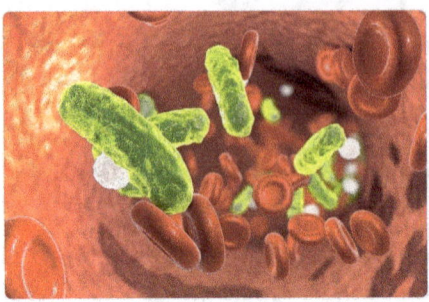

The infection may spread to other parts of the immune system is weak. In widespread inflammation, the tissue is threatened to be damaged, which may interfere with blood flow around the body. If the blood flow is interrupted, it may cause the blood pressure to drop to dangerously low levels and prevent Oxygen from reaching all the organs and tissues of the body. This may also happen if the infection is severe.

Sources of infection (entry points)

Though Sepsis may be triggered by an infection anywhere in the body, some common sites, such as the lungs, abdomen, pelvis, and urinary tract, may lead to Sepsis.

Spread of Sepsis by extensive use of AVF and CVC

There are three common vascular accesses for Hemodialysis. These are:

- Autologous arteriovenous fistulas (AVFs)
- Prosthetic grafts (AVGs)
- Central venous catheters (CVCs)

Of these three most common options, professionals highly recommend the AVF as the vascular access for Hemodialysis. This is because of lower morbidity and mortality rates compared to the other two options. Extensive use of AVF has the least risk of spreading Sepsis.

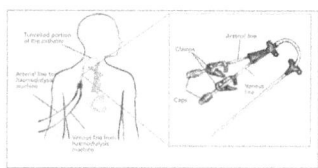

Starting dialysis via a CVC does not cause an increase in the risk of death. Patients are more likely to die by dialyzing by a catheter instead of an AVF. In contrast, fistulas have a lower risk of infection when compared to CVCs.

To avoid fistula malfunctioning and ensure high patency, AVFs have the potential to last longer as compared to catheters. They are also linked with a shorter length of stay when patients are admitted for complications related to vascular access.

CHAPTER FOUR:
DIALYSIS-RELATED MATTERS

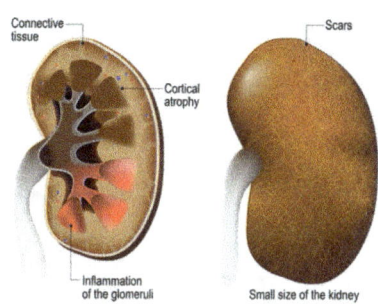

Glomerulonephritis (GN) is one of the causes of Kidney Failure and a condition that causes damage to the filters in the kidneys. Glomerulonephritis is a condition that causes inflammation in the tiny filters present in the kidney. If the inflammation continues unabated for a long time, it may damage the kidneys. This condition can be acute or chronic, which it may have an abrupt or gradual onset. This condition may manifest on its own or, in some cases, be due to other diseases. Possible examples of other diseases causing the onset of Glomerulonephritis are lupus and diabetes.

So, Glomerulonephritis, a type of kidney disease potentially damaging the tiny filters in the kidney known as glomeruli, must be taken seriously. There are different reasons this disease may occur, and possible causes include infections and issues with the immune system. Abuse of drugs like marijuana and heroin is also a possible suspect, as is nicotine. Artificial additives and preservatives used in foods, such as MSG, sodium nitrites/nitrates, artificial food colorings, high fructose corn syrup, artificial sweeteners, or sugar, may also cause this issue.

In some cases, Glomerulonephritis is mild, and the issue may be resolved independently. In other cases, it may persist long and lead to severe consequences, such as kidney failure or other complications. Hence, looking out for its symptoms is essential.

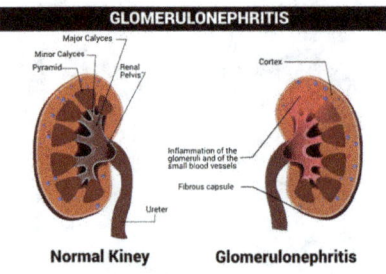

Glomerulonephritis is also addressed as GN or simply glomerular disease.

The critical function of glomeruli

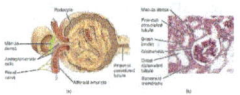

The tiny filtering units in the kidney are known as glomeruli. These are made up of tiny blood vessels or capillaries. They help the body filter blood by removing water and extra fluid. They are thus involved in the process that produces urine. Hence, the health of glomeruli is vital to the human body because of its essential function.

How is Glomerulonephritis classified?

If this condition has a sudden onset, it is known as acute Glomerulonephritis. In case, it is a gradual process that lasts for a considerable time. It is known as chronic Glomerulonephritis. The condition may manifest as an acute attack, following which a chronic condition may appear after some years. Acute Glomerulonephritis may go away independently, while chronic Glomerulonephritis requires treatment.

Causes of Glomerulonephritis

The reasons behind Glomerulonephritis may be unknown, but experts have identified a few causes. Genetics may play a role in this condition, which may be hereditary. However, this rarely happens. A disease known as anti-GBM, a group of diseases, may also be the culprit affecting the lungs and kidneys. An infection inside the heart valves known as endocarditis may also cause Glomerulonephritis. Other issues include strep throat, HIV, or hepatitis C. Issues with the immune system may also herald the onset of Glomerulonephritis. An example is lupus. In rare cases, diseases that cause inflammation of the blood vessels may also cause this condition.

Symptoms of Glomerulonephritis

The problem with Glomerulonephritis is that the patients may not experience any signs or symptoms. Possible symptoms are mentioned below:

- Blood in the urine. This may result in the color of the urine turning brown, red, or pink

- Signs of fatigue, nausea, or a rash
- High blood pressure
- Shortness of breath
- Joint or abdominal pain
- Urinating less or more than normal
- Swelling in the leg or face
- Foamy urine

Experts usually urge caution and recommend seeing a healthcare professional if one or more of these symptoms are present.

Diagnosing Glomerulonephritis

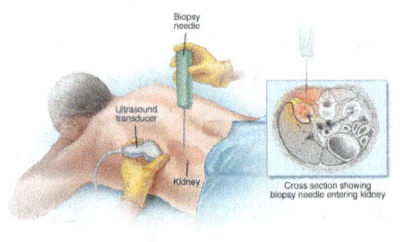

As in any other disease, the first possible clues are the symptoms. However, symptoms are not always present. Since protein and blood cells in the urine are possible signs, blood tests will help a healthcare professional diagnose the disease and determine how much harm has been caused to the kidneys. In other cases, a kidney biopsy, a form of test, may be required. This test requires a piece of the kidney to be removed with the help of a special needle and examined by a microscope. A biopsy is very useful as it will help the doctor devise the best treatment plan for the patient.

Preventing Glomerulonephritis

This is a difficult task and will remain so until more details are found about the causes behind Glomerulonephritis. However, a few precautionary steps can be adopted to prevent the onset of this disease. Following good hygiene is essential. Safe sex and avoiding unprotected sex and drugs that may cause diseases such as hepatitis and HIV is crucial. These diseases are known to lead to Glomerulonephritis.

Those who suffer from chronic Glomerulonephritis must control their blood pressure. Consuming less protein may help. This will help slow down the damage being caused to the kidney. It is also essential to plan your diet; assistance may be sought from a dietician, especially a renal dietician.

Here are a few steps you can adopt to prevent its onset:

- Consuming healthy and unprocessed foods
- Controlling BP with a low salt diet and being regular with exercise and medication
- Prevent infections through reasonable hygienic measures
- Avoiding the use of needles for drugs and tattoos
- Seeing the doctor for infections like strep throat

Treatment options available for Glomerulonephritis

Acute Glomerulonephritis may go away on its own. In some cases, temporary treatment may be required. This involves using an artificial kidney machine to remove the extra fluid. It will also help control high blood pressure and prevent possible kidney failure. Though antibiotics help treat diseases resulting from bacterial infection, they still cannot be used to treat acute Glomerulonephritis.

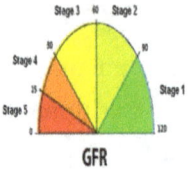

If the illness progresses rapidly, the patient may need high doses of medicines that may harm the immune system. A unique blood filtering process may be required, known as plasmapheresis. This process is necessary to remove the harmful proteins that may be present in your bloodstream.

The problem with chronic Glomerulonephritis is that no specific treatment is available now. Experts recommend a few steps in such cases. These are:

- Eating less protein
- Eating less salt and potassium
- Controlling BP
- Treating swelling with diuretics (water pills)
- Intake of calcium supplements
- Avoiding abuse of drugs, especially the ones that require the use of needles
- Reducing or eliminating the consumption of food containing artificial additives and preservatives. Examples include avoiding foods containing sodium nitrites/nitrates, artificial food colorings, high fructose corn syrup, artificial sweetener
- Using natural or organic preservatives. Examples are natural extracts, such as vinegar and garlic.

The doctor may prescribe a few medications to treat this condition. These medicines are intended to reduce morbidity and prevent complications from arising. For this purpose, medicines such as angiotensin-converting enzyme inhibitors (ACEIs) and angiotensin II receptor blockers (ARBs) may be used. Other options include calcium channel blockers, diuretics, alpha-adrenergic agonists, and beta-adrenergic blockers.

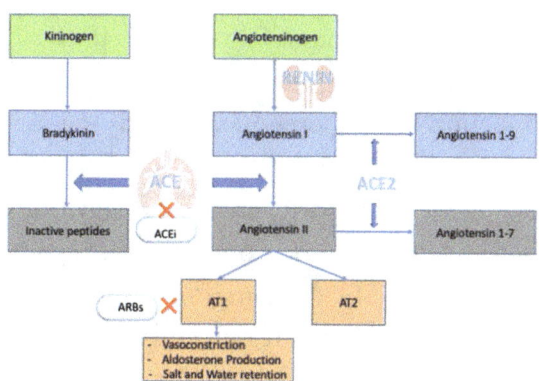

Complications of Glomerulonephritis

Since Glomerulonephritis affects nephrons and their ability to filter the blood effectively, it may result in different complications. This is because it accumulates waste and toxins in the blood and loses red blood cells and proteins. It also results in the poor regulation of minerals and nutrients required by the body.

Glomerulonephritis may result in acute kidney failure. This refers to the sudden and rapid decline of kidney function. It is related to the infectious cause of Glomerulonephritis. In this scenario, the accumulated waste and fluids must be treated and removed immediately, or the condition may result in death. It requires the use of dialysis. However, the good news is that the kidneys will start functioning again after recovery.

Another complication of Glomerulonephritis is chronic kidney disease. This happens if there is prolonged inflammation that may eventually result in kidney function decline due to long-term damage. It may also advance to the end stage of kidney disease. This will then require treatment through dialysis or a kidney transplant.

Another possible complication of Glomerulonephritis is high blood pressure resulting from damage to the glomeruli. The damage occurs due to inflammation of the glomeruli and leads to increased BP.

In some cases, Glomerulonephritis may eventually lead to nephrotic syndrome. In this condition, the urine contains high of blood protein and too little in the bloodstream. Protein is crucial as it plays a role in regulating both cholesterol levels and fluids. If the body's protein levels drop, it will result in high cholesterol and blood pressure. It will also cause swelling of the different parts of the body, such as hands, feet, face, and abdomen. The most concerning part about this condition is that, in rare cases, it leads to a blood clot in the kidney blood vessel.

The diet that helps with acute Glomerulonephritis

- Lean meat (fish, poultry)
- Beans (chickpeas, soybeans)
- Peanuts
- Butter
- Fruits (apples, watermelons, bananas, oranges, pears)
- Vegetables (tomato, potato, lettuce)
- Rice
- Cereals
- Snacks containing little salt
- Low sodium diet

- Foods containing preservatives
- Using the natural method of freezing, heating, and controlling moisture to preserve foods

Illicit use of drugs and Glomerulonephritis

Several renal disorders stem from drug abuse. Drug abuse is associated with numerous medical complications, including Glomerulonephritis. Complications from drug abuse include post-infectious Glomerulonephritis and hepatitis-related Glomerulonephritis. Both these conditions develop in intravenous drug addicts.

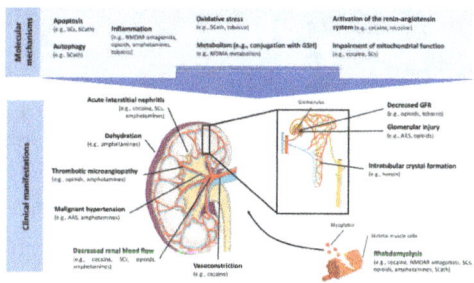

It is important to note that drugs may lead to inflammatory changes in the glomerulus. The inflammation can also occur in the renal tubular cells and the surrounding interstitium. Possible complications resulting from these issues are renal scarring and fibrosis.

Uremic toxins and health concerns

Kidneys perform many functions, and one such important function is to eliminate the waste products and toxins that accumulate in the bloodstream due to the body's different metabolic processes.

A normal kidney will eliminate all these solutes that are harmful to the human body. This will ensure that the blood and tissue concentrations are kept at relatively low levels. If these toxins are left untreated, they may harm our health. The toxic retention leads to uremia in patients, as observed in patients who suffer from advanced chronic kidney disease and end-stage renal disease.

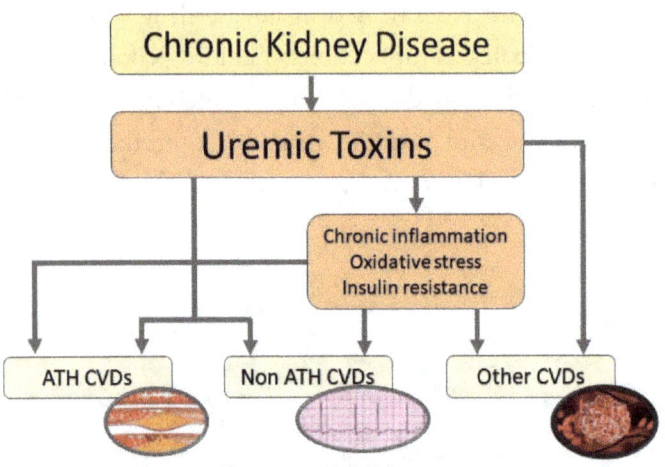

Uremic toxins are classified into three categories. In classic taxonomy, the uremic retention compounds are known as:

- Small solutes
- Middle molecules
- and protein-bound toxins

Uremic toxins may be defined as those substances, whether organic or inorganic, that have accumulated in the body fluids. This typically happens in patients with acute or chronic kidney disease. It also affects those who have impaired kidney function. These conditions collectively manifest in uremic syndrome. It is easier to classify these conditions based on physicochemical properties, mainly molecular size, protein binding, and organ tropism. A significant number of uremic toxins result from protein metabolism. Factors such as colonic microbiota and enterohepatic circulation mainly influence these. Uremic toxins are generated because of the diet composition, especially by the animal and vegetable proteins in the diet. These factors influence the generation of uremic toxins. Research has proven that most of the low and middle-molecular-weight toxins are removed from the bloodstream through glomerular filtration. In this regard, the protein-bound uremic toxins use tubular secretion as a possible removal pathway.

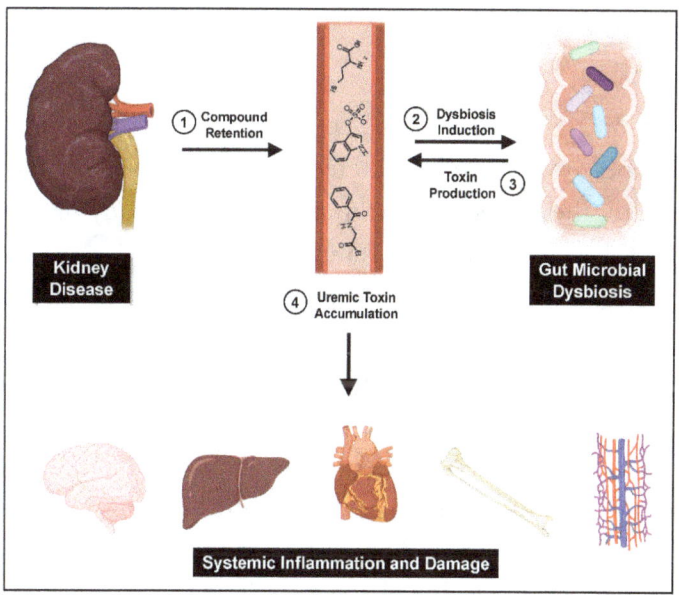

Dialysis has proven to be an efficient means of removing low-molecular-weight uremic toxins. However, dialysis is not very effective in removing the high molecular weight. These are also known as protein-bound uremic toxins.

The past two decades have witnessed a significant interest of medical professionals in forging a close understanding of the uremic syndrome. The focus has been on uremic toxins' impact on chronic kidney diseases. Uremic toxins may be defined as organic compounds residuals that are not removed from the body naturally and end up accumulating in the bloodstream. This way, they reach the body's organs, such as the kidneys and heart. Currently, the complete details of the uremic toxins are unavailable. However, studies have determined that these toxins increase if the patient suffers from chronic kidney disease. The result is several functional changes in the body.

Uremic toxins and dialysis

Focusing on the protein-bound toxins is essential because, despite dialysis, these toxins are not filtered. The dialysis membrane is not able to filter these protein-bound toxins. Hence, studying their role in patients becomes very important.

Different alternatives have been studied to filter these toxins over the past few years to filter these toxins. One of the alternatives proposed and widely utilized for filtering these toxins is the new type of dialysis. This has been researched in recent years. Examples include high-flux dialysis and also other alternates that utilize different membranes. High flux dialysis uses membranes designed considering the need to remove medium molecules. However, it is essential to mention that the clearance is ineffective in molecules with a molecular mass more significant than 15 (kDa). Examples of such molecules are myoglobulin, 17(kDa),and FGF-23 (32kDa). Studies comparing patients who underwent high-flux Hemodialysis and then medium cut-off (MCO) membrane hemodialysis showed reduced middle molecular mass molecule levels. The myoglobulin and β2-microglobulin were found to be significantly reduced in the first and last sessions when the MCO dialyzers were used in contrast to the high-flux dialyzers. This suggests that this method is effective in lowering the levels of uremic toxin.

Studies have also recently established that using the MCO membrane can significantly reduce albumin serum levels within three months. However, these studies have not concluded whether the serum albumin level decrease is definite.

Uremic toxins and altered mental status

Different types of neuropsychiatric conditions are found in patients who suffer from chronic kidney disease. These include severe mental health conditions like depression, anxiety, and cognitive impairment. These conditions heavily affect the patient's overall health and deteriorate their quality of life. At times, these conditions may also increase the risk of hospitalization and cause higher mortality rates. The past few years have witnessed numerous efforts being made to study the impact of such conditions and the possible links between chronic kidney disease and neuropsychiatric disorders.

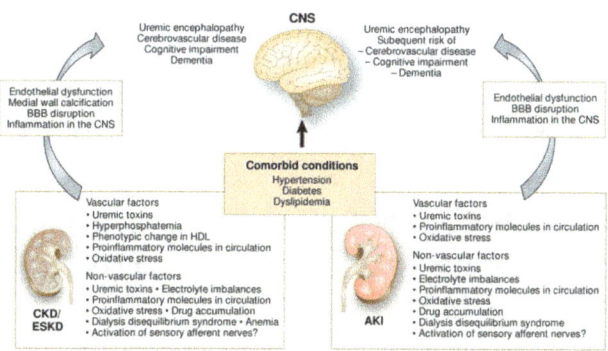

The central point of the outcome of all such studies establishes the link between the rate of cerebrovascular disease and the accumulated uremic toxins in patients who suffer from chronic kidney disease. Studies have demonstrated this meaningful connection but have failed to establish a close link or direct association between the various vascular risk factors known worldwide, such as diabetes and hypertension, and chronic kidney disease-related cognitive deficits. This suggests that other factors may be a part of the pathophysiology common to renal and neuropsychiatric diseases. This fact is supported by neuropsychiatric comorbidities in pediatric patients with chronic kidney disease.

Several studies conducted in the past have established a link between a decrease in renal function with cognitive impairment. It has been proven that for every decrease of 15 ml/min/1.73 m2 in glomerular filtration rate (GFR), an estimated decline in cognitive function is comparable to that of a 3-year aging. Hence, chronic kidney disease turns out to be an established risk factor that contributes to cognitive decline.

Psychiatric disorders are not uncommon for those who suffer from chronic kidney disease. The likelihood of hospitalizations for psychiatric disorders, such as anxiety, depression, and substance abuse, is almost three times higher for chronic disease patients than for patients suffering from other chronic diseases. The problem does not end here, as the resulting cognitive impairment or other psychiatric disorders lead to low life quality in patients suffering from chronic kidney disease. As mentioned earlier in this chapter, chronic kidney disease leads to elevated levels of uremic toxins in the body.

Uremic toxins inflict neuronal damage, which has far more repercussions than hemodynamic factors or lipid metabolism. Uremic toxins levels in the body increase as the renal clearance function deteriorate, leading to many severe effects, from systemic inflammation to cardiac failure and Anemia to other issues like anorexia, immune dysfunction, cognitive impairment, and neurological damage. Another effect of the high levels of uremic toxins present in the body of chronic kidney disease patients is that it passes through the blood-brain barrier, known as BBB. It then causes cognitive dysfunction and neurodegeneration. The risks of cognitive impairments in such patients are increased due to different uremic toxins. These include para-cresyl sulfate (PCS), fibroblast growth factor 23 (FGF23) phosphate, and indoxyl sulfate (IS). It has also been established that the brain's monoaminergic system is susceptible to uremic neurotoxins.

p-Cresyl sulfate (PCS)   Indoxyl sulfate (IS)

High sugar diet and the role of fungi, bacteria, and viruses in increasing C-reactive protein

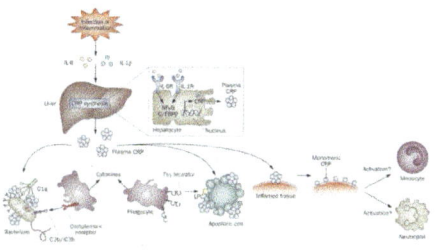

CRP (c-reactive protein) is a protein made by the liver. The main reason why the liver tends to release more CRP into the bloodstream is in case of inflammation in the body. High levels of CRP are a severe medical concern as it indicates an underlying health condition causing inflammation in the body. An average person without any medical condition will have low levels of c-reactive protein in their blood.

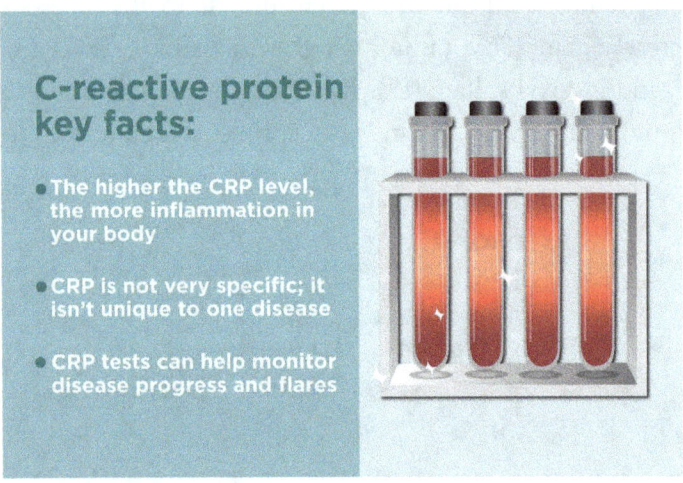

If the CRP test results point towards high levels of CRP, it indicates acute inflammation in the body resulting from infection or an injury. In some cases, it may also be due to chronic disease.

A high-sugar diet allows the fungi, bacteria, and viruses to bind in the sugar on the cell's surface, increasing the C-reactive protein and thus causing infections. The metabolic pathway process through which this occurs is known as Gluconeogenesis. In this process, these microorganisms produce more sugar in the blood, which renders the patient Hyperglycemic. This is a severe condition that causes altered mental status. These pathogens cause an increase in glucose levels. This is the precursor to many diseases, such as DM, Rheumatoid Arthritis, and Alzheimer's.

The link between high blood sugar and high CRP

Doctors use C-reactive protein as a sensitive marker of systemic inflammation to determine an individual's health. Records suggest this condition increases in patients diagnosed with type 2 diabetes mellitus. CRP levels have also been high in people who demonstrated the features of metabolic syndrome or were suffering from cardiovascular disease.

A CRP test's moderately elevated levels of c-reactive protein range from 1.0 to 10.0 milligrams per deciliter (mg/dL). This range may result from conditions that cause systemic inflammation, such as systemic lupus erythematosus, autoimmune conditions, and rheumatoid arthritis.

Effect of sugar on C-reactive protein?

C-reactive protein has a positive relationship with sugar intake while not associated with the intake of minerals, vitamins, fruit, and vegetables.

As mentioned above, the level of CRP increases following inflammation in the body. The levels undergo an increase due to inflammatory proteins known as cytokines. Proteins, known as acute phase reactants, increase when there is inflammation.

Gluconeogenesis occurs due to the synthesis of new glucose from non-carbohydrate precursors. This occurs when the glucose consumed from the diet is insufficient to meet the body's demands. This process is integral to regulating the acid-base balance and amino acid metabolism.

If the blood glucose levels drop significantly, the body responds by releasing the hormones epinephrine and glucagon. Releasing these hormones stimulates glycogenolysis, restoring blood glucose levels to normal levels. Patients diagnosed with type 1 diabetes are at risk as they may suffer from losing the ability to secrete glucagon and epinephrine. This has the potential for repercussions as it may lead hypoglycemia.

Why treating hyperglycemia is important

A failure to treat hyperglycemia could lead to a condition known as ketoacidosis (diabetic coma). Ketoacidosis occurs when the body lacks sufficient insulin. A lack of insulin means the body cannot use glucose as fuel. Consequently, the body breaks down fats as a source of energy.

Hyperglycemia leads to altered mental status

Acute hyperglycemia has been proven to cause changes in mental health. It alters the mood state and leads to an impairment in cognitive performance in diabetes mellitus patients. Patients diagnosed with diabetes mellitus experience delirium when undergoing ketoacidosis or hypoglycemia.

Here is how hyperglycemia affects the mental status of an individual

There is a close association between diabetic patients and those with higher blood glucose levels (hyperglycemia) with anger or sadness. Dips in blood sugar dips (hypoglycemia) are linked with nervousness. However, others, apart from those with diabetes, face the threat of mood fluctuations due to blood sugar fluctuations.

High blood sugar is closely associated with increased protein pieces known as beta-amyloid in medical terminology. These protein pieces may clump together, causing them to be stuck between the nerve cells in the brain, resulting in blocked signals, a close feature of Alzheimer's.

Among other possible conditions that may be caused due to high blood sugar is Rheumatoid Arthritis.

The link between hyperglycemia and dementia

For patients who suffer from hypoglycemia or hyperglycemia, the risk of dementia is six times higher than for those with regular blood sugar. Research suggests that severe glycemic cases negatively impact the brain, implying that these conditions increase the risk of dementia in older adults with type 1 diabetes.

CRP test

This test helps find or monitor inflammation caused in the body due to acute and chronic conditions.

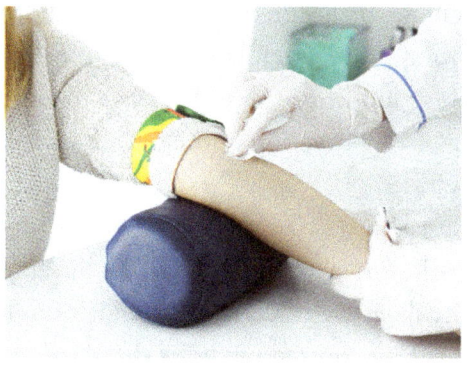

This test is required in case of symptoms of a bacterial infection. These include fever or chills, increased breathing or heart rate, and nausea and vomiting.

A CRP test is also necessary if the individual is suspected to suffer from a chronic condition causing inflammation.

The levels of CRP rise and fall based on the level of inflammation in the body. In case of a fall in CRP levels, it implies that the treatment is effective or that the individual may be healing independently. In case of an earlier diagnosis of either an infection or a chronic disease-causing inflammation, a CRP test may be required for monitoring the condition and devising future treatment plans.

Role of pectin in improving blood sugar and fat levels and promoting healthy body weight

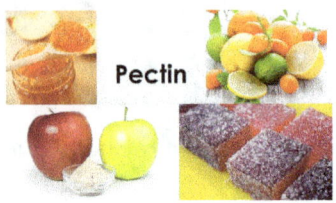

Pectin is found in fruits and vegetables, such as pears, apples, guavas, plums, oranges, and other citrus fruits. It is a soluble fiber that offers many valuable benefits to the body.

One main advantage of pectin is that it improves blood sugar and fat levels. According to research conducted on mice, pectin has the potential to lower blood sugar levels. It leads to an improvement in the blood-sugar-related function of the hormone. It helps in managing type 2 diabetes.

Pectin also helps improve blood fat levels by binding itself with the cholesterol in the digestive tract, preventing it from being absorbed. This lowers the risk of contracting heart disease.

Pectin also promotes a healthy body weight. This is because research has concluded that an increase in fiber intake leads to a decrease in the risk of becoming overweight and obese. This impact is observed because fiber is filling and also due to high-fiber foods being mostly lower in calories than other low-fiber foods.

Research on animals has concluded that pectin supplements promote weight loss and fat burn.

Adding pectin to your diet

An easy way to increase pectin intake is to consume foods high in pectin fiber, like apples. Almost all fruits and vegetables contain some pectin.

A word of caution is to refrain from most jams and jellies. Though these are made from pectin, this fiber is not recommended because they contain only small amounts of fiber and high sugar and calories.

Hypoxia and its benefit to bacterial and fungal pathogen infections

Infections, such as the ones caused by bacterial and fungal pathogens, benefit significantly from Hypoxia. This process allows these microorganisms to consume Oxygen through respiration. This process diminishes the antimicrobial activities of the macrophages and neutrophils in the human body's immune system. Since these activities depend on Oxygen, Hypoxia significantly impacts the production of reactive oxygen species (ROS).

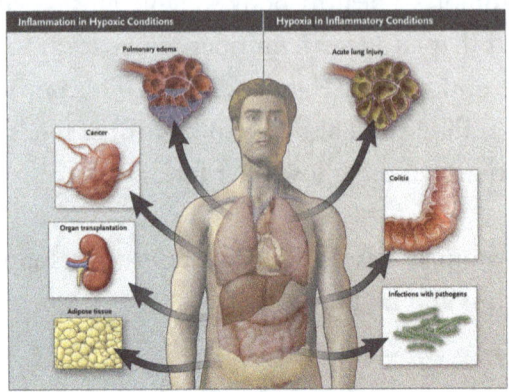

Regarding immune modulatory, besides its antimicrobial activity, ROS is also the precursor to the progression of inflammatory diseases. This occurs due to the increased biological structures and pro-inflammatory cytokines.

Different infectious disease studies have concluded that pathogens stand to benefit from Hypoxia. Aerobic pathogens refer to bacteria that find a way to grow and live in the presence of Oxygen. Since bacteria lack intracellular compartments (organelles), cellular respiration occurs in the cytoplasm and at the plasma membrane. Aerobic respiration utilizes Oxygen in the process.

Some aerobic bacteria use aerobic respiration, such as obligate aerobes, facultative aerobes, microaerophiles, and aerotolerant aerobes.

Either surgical drainage or debridement treats the aerobic infection. Antibiotics may be used to treat certain infections caused by bacteria. However, some bacterial infections may get treated without antibiotics.

CHAPTER FIVE:
INFLAMMATION AND PAIN

Inflammation: An Overview

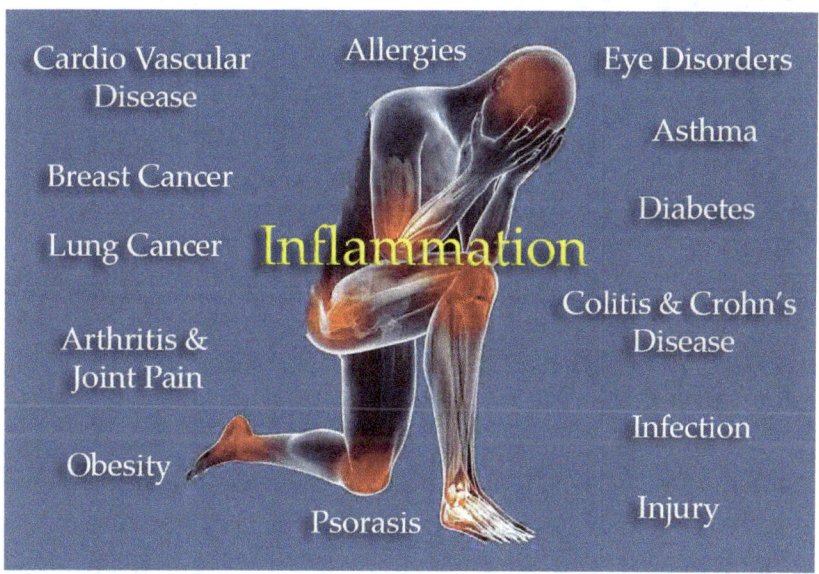

Inflammation plays an essential role in the body's defense mechanism. It is crucial for the healing process. Following an injury or detection of an intruder inside the body, such as pathogens, the body launches its biological response to eliminate the threat. The foreign intruder can be any foreign body, from a thorn to an irritant to a 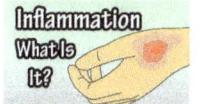 pathogen. Pathogens include foreign bodies, such as viruses, bacteria, or other organisms, that are involved in causing infections.

The body's immune system sends out its first responders in response to an injury or an intruder, such as bacteria. These are the inflammatory cells and cytokines. Cytokines are substances that stimulate additional inflammatory cells. This activates an inflammatory response that leads to the trapping of bacteria and other intruders. It also starts the healing process in which the injured tissues are healed. This eventually results in pain, redness, bruising, or swelling.

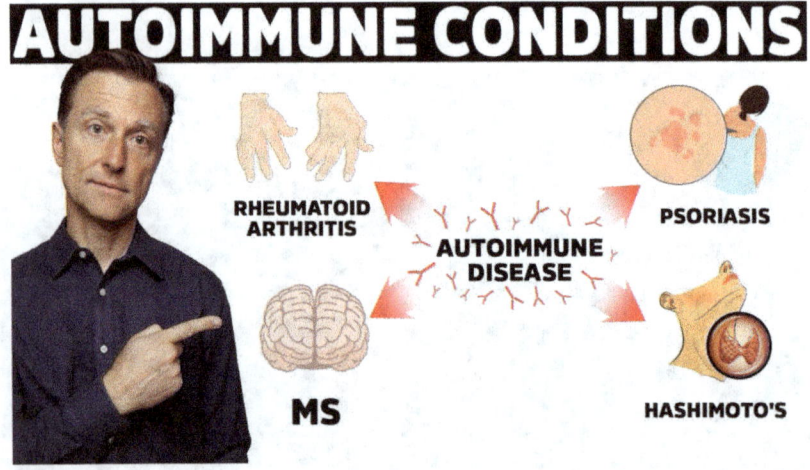

Autoimmune diseases have an essential connection with inflammation. At times, the body may mistakenly perceive its tissues or cells as harmful to itself. This brings about a reaction that eventually causes autoimmune diseases. An example is type 1 diabetes. Experts opine that inflammation is responsible for chronic diseases, such as type 2 diabetes, obesity, and heart diseases. Metabolic syndrome is yet another example of a chronic disease caused by inflammation. The bodies of those who suffer from such conditions have high levels of inflammatory markers.

The Inflammatory Marker (Measuring Inflammation)

In case of inflammation in the body, there will be elevated levels of substances called biomarkers. An important example of a biomarker known to experts is C-reactive protein (CRP), discussed in the previous chapter. The CRP test helps doctors assess the CRP levels in the body and hence the inflammation level.

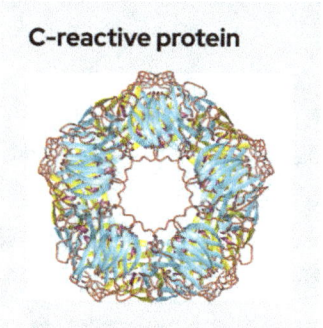

An important point to note is that the CRP levels are higher in aged people and those with some conditions like obesity and cancer. The CRP levels are also influenced by the diet an individual consumes and the nature of the exercise.

Types of inflammation

Experts divide inflammation into two types, known as acute and chronic inflammation.

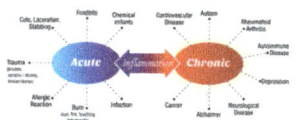

Acute inflammation

An injury or an illness may cause short-term inflammation, also known as acute inflammation. This type of inflammation presents five key signs.

- Pain
- Redness
- Loss of function
- Swelling
- Heat

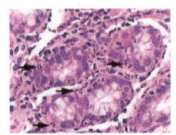

The pain may be continuous or felt when the individual touches the affected part of the body. The redness occurs due to increased blood supply to the capillaries of the affected area. Since inflammation causes difficulty in moving the affected area, such as the joint, it is classified as a loss of function. The swelling occurs because of a condition known as edema due to the buildup of fluids. Heat is an essential sign of acute inflammation as the affected area faces an increased blood flow.

However, it must be noted that these signs may be absent at times, and the inflammation may be regarded as 'silent.' Such an individual may feel unwell and feelings of fatigue. Fever is also a possible symptom.

The duration of these symptoms is usually short-lived, and it may last only a few days. However, the subacute form of inflammation may last longer and span 2 to 6 weeks.

Several reactions are triggered when a body detects damage to a part of the body or invasion by pathogens. An injury, infection, or exposure to a foreign substance may cause acute inflammation. It may lead to plasma proteins accumulating on the affected tissues, causing fluid buildup and swelling.

The body may also respond by releasing white blood cells called neutrophils, also known as leukocyte, that moves on to the affected area. Leukocytes are essential as they are equipped with specific molecules that help fight pathogens. The body also undergoes a change in which the small blood vessels enlarge, allowing the leukocytes and the plasma proteins to access the injury site easily.

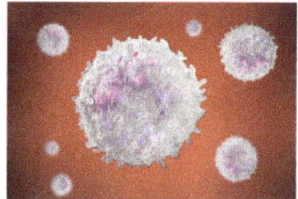

It usually depends on the cause. It may take a few hours or even days for the body to indicate signs of acute inflammation. Here are a few examples of infections and other factors that cause acute inflammation.

- An ingrown toenail
- Sore throat
- Physical trauma
- Acute bronchitis
- Wound
- Appendicitis

Chronic inflammation

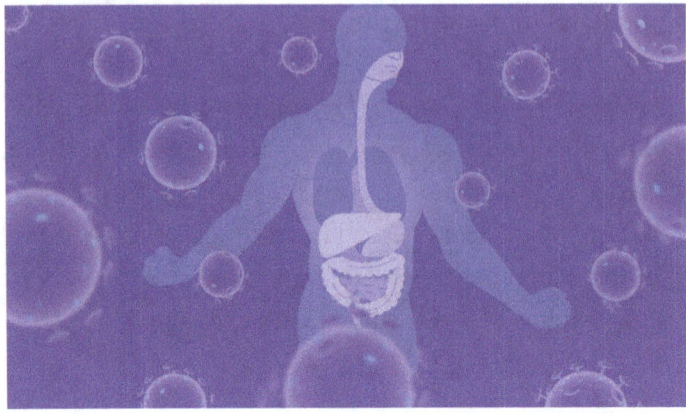

This form of inflammation continues for a more extended period than acute inflammation. It may last for many months and even persist for years. It is known to be linked to various diseases. These could be:

- Allergies
- Arthritis
- Joint diseases
- Cardiovascular diseases
- Psoriasis
- Diabetes
- Rheumatoid arthritis

Such symptoms cause pain and fatigue, but the nature depends on the type of disease.

Chronic inflammation develops due to several factors. Sensitive individuals may develop inflammation when their bodies sense something is not present. This usually involves an allergy developed due to hypersensitivity to an external trigger. Exposure to an irritant for a long time may also lead to inflammation. An example is exposure to an industrial chemical. At times the immune system of individuals may mistakenly perceive a normal healthy tissue as foreign and attack it. This leads to an autoimmune disorder, such as in the case of psoriasis.

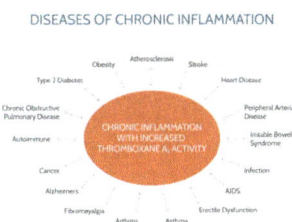

Autoinflammatory diseases may affect the functioning of the immune system. This happens due to a genetic factor that affects the immune system. An example is Behcet's disease.

Another probable cause of chronic inflammation is when an individual fails to recover from acute inflammation.

Nociceptors

The infection caused by pathogens triggers pain in the body. The pain is detected by nociceptors, which are sensory receptors responsible for detecting signals from damaged body tissues. They may also indirectly respond if chemicals are released from the damaged tissue.

Nociceptors in brief

As mentioned above, these pain receptors exist in all body parts as free nerve endings. They are found everywhere, from skin and muscles to joints and bones. Their play a crucial role in how an individual feels and responds to pain.

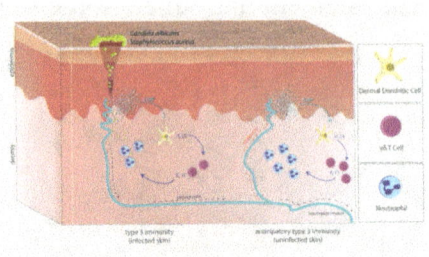

The primary function of these free nerve endings is to respond to damage caused in any part of the body. This response is from signals transmitted to the spinal cord and the brain. Take, for example, the case of pain in your finger. If you stub your finger, this will activate the nociceptors in the skin that will send a signal to the brain. This signal will be transmitted via the peripheral nerves to the spinal cord. This is how pain, in all cases, is messaged.

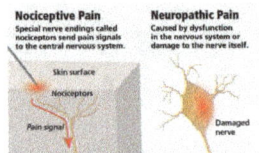

Different classes of Nociceptors

Nociceptors are classified based on the type of stimuli they respond to. Here are the different classes:

Thermal

These are the nociceptors that respond to fluctuations in temperature, like extremely hot or cold. If you touch a hot cup, then this will activate the nociceptors.

Mechanical Nociceptors

These are the ones that respond to an intense strain or a stretch of a body part. An example is when you pull a hamstring. If the tendon muscles stretch beyond their capacity, the nociceptors will be stimulated, which will cause them to send pain signals to the brain.

Chemical Nociceptors

If chemicals are released from tissue damage or the body comes in contact with external chemicals, these chemical nociceptors will respond to the threat.

Silent Nociceptors

Examples of silent nociceptors are nerve endings located in internal organs. These nociceptors need to be activated before they can respond. This occurs when tissue inflammation results from a response to chemical, mechanical or thermal stimuli.

How pain is felt (The transmission of pain)

The above nociceptors were classified based on the type of stimuli they respond to. However, some experts may also classify Nociceptors based on how fast they transmit pain signals. The nerve fiber type, known as the axon in the nociceptors, determines the speed with which nociceptors communicate pain.

Two different types of nerve fibers exist in the nociceptors. The first type is called A fiber axon. These fibers have a fatty protective sheath on all sides known as myelin. Myelin allows nerve signals to travel rapidly to transmit pain signals. The nerve signals are also known as action potentials.

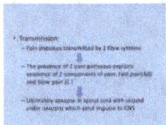

The other type of nerve fiber is known as C fiber axons. These are not surrounded by myelin and transmit nerve signals at a slower pace.

Since there is a difference in the transmission speed between A and C fibers, the spinal cord first receives pain signals from fiber A. In an acute injury, the individual will receive pain from the A and C fibers in two phases.

The different phases of pain perception

Following an injury, such as a cut on your finger, the A fibers are activated, which causes the individual to experience pain that prickles and is sharp. This pain is not intense but is felt immediately following a painful stimulus. Experts call this the first phase of pain, also called fast pain.

The next phase, known as the second path of pain, comes following the activation of the C fibers. In this phase, the individual experiences pain that is intense and has a burning sensation. It persists even after the stimulus has stopped.

Since the C fibers carry the burning pain, experts now know why there is a short delay before an individual feels pain following a painful external stimulus such as touching a hot pot. Another aching or sore pain also occurs due to the C fibers. It comes from organs within the body. Examples are sore muscles and stomach pain.

The role of Manuka honey in fighting disease-causing bacteria and alleviating inflammation

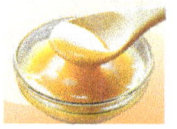

Manuka honey is produced by bees pollinating on the tea tree, classified as a Leptospermum scoparium, a native of Australia and New Zealand. The reason for interest in this type of honey is its properties that offer various benefits, including aiding the healing of wounds.

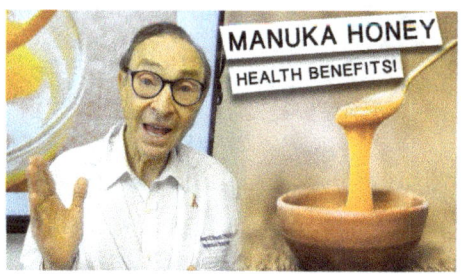

With both antioxidant and antibiotic properties, Manuka honey helps reduce inflammation and fight bacteria that cause disease in the human body. It is a valuable product that helps the body fight off conditions such as joint pain or inflamed arthritis, wounds, ulcers, and burns.

Generally speaking, honey is used worldwide and almost in every culture to prevent infection. It is also used to improve wound healing. Recently, Manuka honey has been recognized as a valuable source of fighting bacteria and reducing inflammation. Having demonstrated to be potentially successful in alleviating several conditions, it has potent antibacterial and anti-inflammatory therapeutic properties. This has paved the way for Manuka honey to be used in different wound dressings. It is also consumed for its anti-inflammatory and antioxidant effects.

Research on Manuka honey has identified it as a potential source of biomaterial additive with promising results in reducing acute inflammation.

Hydrogen peroxide is the reason why honey provides antibiotic quality. However, some types, like Manuka honey, are essential as they also offer unique antibacterial qualities.

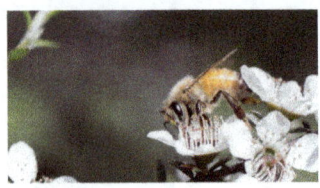

Manuka Honey is important because it has an antibacterial component known as methylglyoxal (MGO). MGO is formed due to a compound in Manuka honey known as dihydroxyacetone (DHA). DHA is found in a high concentration in the nectar of Manuka flowers.

Manuka honey is essential because it helps protect the body from damage caused by bacteria. It also aids in tissue repair that has been damaged by infection. It also activates an anti-inflammatory response that is vital in easing pain and inflammation.

Pus: An Overview

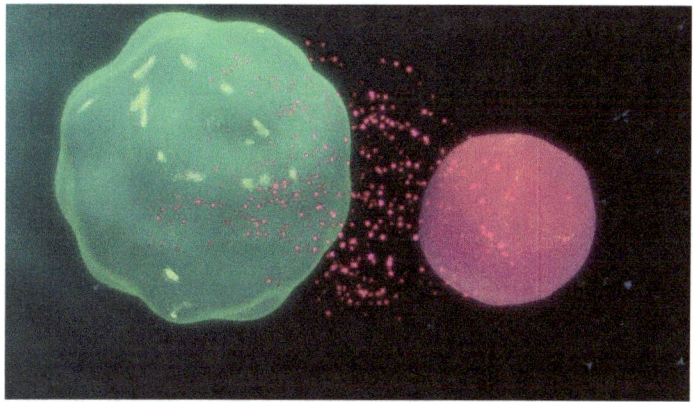

Pus is a thick fluid that forms when dead tissues, cells, and bacteria accumulate in one place. Pus is produced when the body is fighting an infection. Typically, such infections are caused by bacteria. The color of the pus varies depending on the type of infection and the location where it occurs. It may be odorless or may cause a foul smell. Possible colors of pus are white, green, yellow, and brown.

Reasons why pus is formed

Infections that cause pus formation are due to fungi or bacteria entering the body through different parts, such as inhaled droplets from coughing, sneezing, and broken skin. Poor hygiene may also contribute to infection.

After the body has detected an infection, the defense mechanism responds by sending white blood cells known as neutrophils to eliminate the bacteria causing the infection. As these white cells fight the bacteria or fungi, some white cells and tissue would die in the infected area. The dead material then accumulates together, forming the pus.

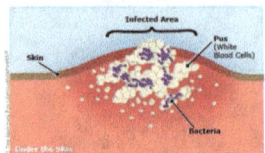

Many types of infections can cause pus formation. Infections caused by bacteria streptococcus pyogenes or staphylococcus aureus commonly form pus. These bacteria contribute to pus formation by releasing toxins that damage the tissue.

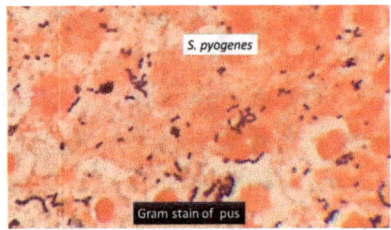

Locations where pus forms

An abscess is a cavity or space where pus forms. This cavity is the result of the breakdown of tissue. These abscesses may form inside the human body or on the skin's surface.

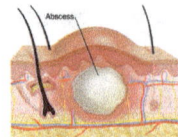

Areas where abscesses may form are the urinary tract, skin, mouth, and eyes. Since some body parts receive greater exposure, they are most susceptible to forming pus following an infection.

Symptoms caused by pus

In case of an infection that causes pus formation, the human body may experience other symptoms. If the infection occurs on the skin surface, the skin around the abscess may turn red and warm. Such areas are usually painful and swollen.

On the other hand, internal abscesses do not demonstrate many visible symptoms. However, flu-like symptoms may be felt. These may manifest in the form of fever, fatigue, and chills.

Such symptoms may also be felt in case of a severe skin infection.

Treating Pus

The treatment of the pus usually depends on the seriousness of the infection that caused its formation. It is easy to treat small abscesses that form on the skin's surface. Appling a wet compress will help drain the pus. The compress must also be warm; applying it a few times for a few minutes will get rid of the pus.

However, it is important not to squeeze the abscess. Though an urge may make the individual feel like a squeeze will help eliminate the issue, it only pushes the pus more deeply into the skin and creates a new open wound. This will then make it vulnerable to forming another infection.

Medical attention is required if the abscess is more profound and more significant. A healthcare professional will remove the pus through a needle that draws out the pus. A small incision may also be necessary to drain the pus. A drainage tube may be inserted to drain the pus in case of a very large abscess that is harder to reach. Additionally, a medicated gauze may also be required.

Deeper infections may require using antibiotics. This is especially true for infections that do not heal.

Reducing the risk of pus

Since some infections are unavoidable, pus formation in such cases will be inevitable. However, a few steps can be taken to reduce the risk of pus formation. As a precautionary move, keep all cuts and wounds clean. They must also be kept dry. Razors should not be shared; new ones should always be used. Avoid the urge to pick pimples.

If an abscess has been formed, it is necessary to avoid its spread. Its spread can be prevented by not sharing towels or bedding. Some experts advise avoiding sharing the communal swimming pools and gym equipment that may touch the abscess. Washing hands in case the hands have touched the abscess is necessary to prevent the spread of infection.

Since pus is a common product of the body's defense mechanism to fight infections, its formation may sometimes be inevitable. The minor infections that cause pus formation, such as the ones on the skin surface, may heal independently without needing treatment. However, severe infections require medical attention. These may involve drainage tubes or the use of antibiotics. If an abscess is not healing, then a doctor should be contacted.

CHAPTER SIX:
CLOTTING PROBLEMS AND DVT IN THE CIRCULATORY SYSTEM

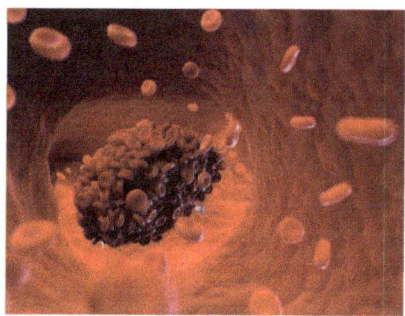

Does dehydration spike blood sugar?

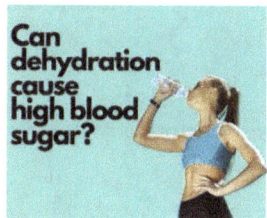

When a body undergoes dehydration, the amount of water in the bloodstream decreases. This leads to the glucose (sugar) levels in the bloodstream becoming more concentrated.

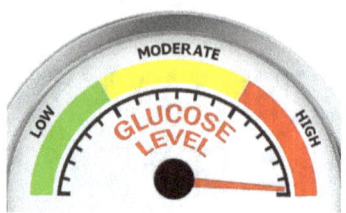

Technically speaking, the sugar levels in the bloodstream remain unchanged, but still, it implies that there would be high blood sugar levels due to the change in sugar to water ratio.

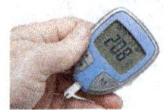

For example, consider the case of maple syrup. It would be best to collect the sap from the trees when making maple syrup. Sap comprises 95% water, while the sugar concentration is only 5%. When you boil the sap, the amount of water is decreased due to evaporation. Hence, the sap becomes more concentrated, resulting in a sweet syrup when put on pancakes. A decrease in water content or less water leads to a higher sugar concentration.

Similarly, the human body needs to maintain adequate water levels in the bloodstream. Maintaining a water vs. glucose ratio ideal for the human body is necessary.

The dangers of dehydration

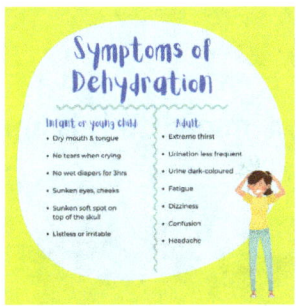

The body is not suited to dehydration. Even mild to moderate levels of dehydration produce negative results. If the weather is hot, an illness like diarrhea or vomiting can increase blood sugar. Intense exercise also produces the same result. In such cases, the blood sugar levels may increase by 50 to 100 mg/dL.

Severe dehydration has more severe consequences and has the potential to be life-threatening. Many factors come into play in such extreme circumstances. This includes concentrated blood sugar levels with fewer electrolytes, sodium, and potassium.

Experts advise that if an individual is suffering from an illness that is causing dehydration or vomiting, which makes it challenging to intake sufficient fluids, then the person should seek urgent medical attention.

In such cases, opting to rehydrate by intaking intravenous fluids or drinking water will help your body reduce blood sugar levels to normal.

Though hydration fluids are essential, following precaution regarding fluids like Gatorade and Pedialyte is still necessary, as they contain sugar.

Treating dehydration immediately is important

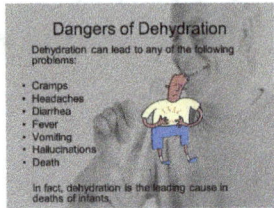

It is important to treat dehydration immediately. If you ignore the issue, severe dehydration may eventually cause the body to suffer from diabetic ketoacidosis. The body may also face other life-threatening conditions in case of severe dehydration.

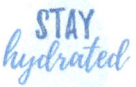

Thus, dehydration increases the glucose concentration in the bloodstream leading to high blood sugar levels because the sugar-to-H2O ratio becomes imbalanced.

Impact of blood sugar on blood viscosity and changes caused to blood consistency

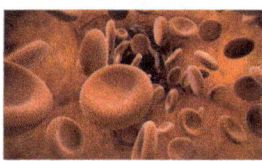

Blood sugar has a direct effect on blood viscosity and has the potential to change the composition of blood and hamper its functioning. A high glucose concentration in the bloodstream means the blood consistency becomes thicker. Different factors linked to the blood composition directly or indirectly affect the blood viscosity. Also known as hemorheological factors, they have an important role in the pathogenesis of different disorders. One of the critical factors that affect blood viscosity is glucose. If glucose levels increase in the body, it leads to an increase in resistance in the blood flow.

Studies have concluded that an increase in the blood glucose mean value from 00 to 400 mg/dL will cause the blood viscosity to increase by 25% (r= 0.59, P = .002). This will lead to the blood flow rate decreasing by 20% and also cause the BP to increase.

Among the various factors that experts have found affecting blood viscosity include hematocrit values and plasma fibrinogen levels. Erythrocyte deformability is yet another factor that affects blood viscosity.

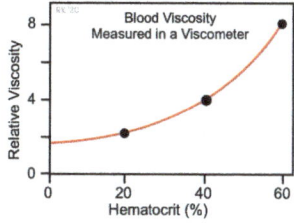

Viscosity of plasma

When studying the viscosity of plasma, it was found that it depends on the concentration of plasma proteins. These plasma proteins are:

- fibrinogen
- α1-globulins
- α2-globulins
- β-globulins
- γ-globulins

Plasma Proteins

Immunoglobulins

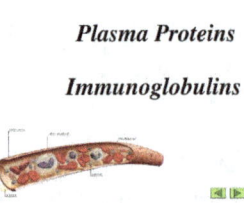

In case the concentration of these proteins increases, they may cause the blood viscosity to increase.

Hyperviscosity

Hyperviscosity syndrome (HVS) is the clinical outcome caused increase in blood viscosity. The effects of hyperviscosity vary from person to person. In case the blood becomes thicker, it will cause poor brain circulation. This condition will lead to various symptoms, such as dizziness, headaches, and confusion. Sometimes, the individuals may also experience shortness of breath or blurry vision.

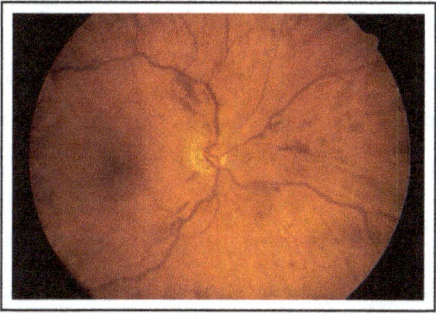

High glucose levels can also damage the blood vessels and impact the circulatory system severely. This increases in blood viscosity and affects the heart and blood flow through the formation of clots.

Detailed information on blood clots is presented below in the Hypercoagulability section.

Hypocoagulation (When blood fails to clot normally)

Hypocoagulation is a condition in which the blood fails to clot normally. It is a severe condition and must not be left untreated. This serious disorder may cause hemorrhage, resulting in brain or gastrointestinal bleeding. Some conditions affect the blood's ability to clot normally. These could be thrombocytopenia or a drop in platelet count.

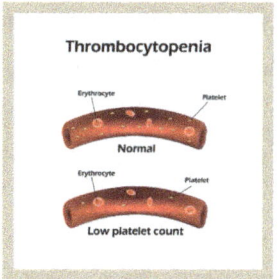

The hypercoagulable state

Owing to one or more predisposing factors, the body enters the hypercoagulable state, also termed thrombophilia. In this condition, there is an increased tendency of the blood to develop blood clots, known as thrombosis. These predisposing factors can be inherited or even acquired. In normal circumstances, a clot is not a negative sign as a blood clot allows the body to heal cuts and injuries.

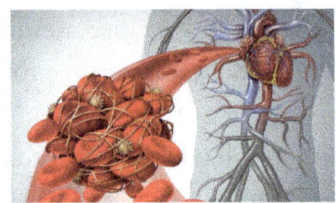

Thromboembolic conditions and deep vein thrombosis

The problem occurs blood clots start developing within blood vessels. This means that people in a hypercoagulable state are prone to developing thromboembolic conditions due to the heightened risk. These conditions could be deep vein thrombosis (pulmonary embolism). Deep vein thrombosis is a medical condition in which a clot develops in one of the deep veins in either the lower or upper limbs. This condition manifests in pain and swelling on the site affected (limb). At times, parts of these venous blood clots tend to break away and end up in the lungs, which leads to a condition known as pulmonary embolism.

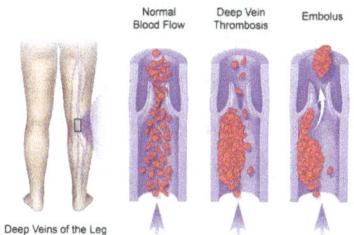

Arterial clots and infarction

There is also the possibility that the arterial clots can travel to other locations. They may end up in organs like the brain, liver, and kidneys. They may also travel to the heart. This may result in the blood flow being cut to these organs, resulting in infarction.

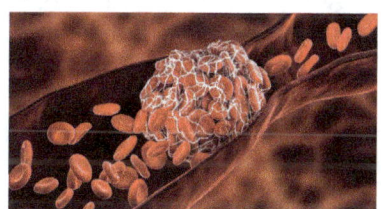

Dehydration and a possible link with insulin resistance

Studies conducted in animals and humans have pointed out hypohydration (low water intake) is closely linked to poor glucose regulation and diabetes. Similar studies also suggest that dehydration may cause an increase in the hormone vasopressin levels in the body. This change causes the kidneys to retain more water. The liver produces blood sugar, so the body's ability to regulate insulin over time is affected.

To add details, it is necessary to know that the hormone Vasopressin is released when the body becomes dehydrated which stimulates the liver to start sugar production in the bloodstream. Experts point out that this link does cause insulin resistance. However, read on to find how there is a close link between the hormone Vasopressin and insulin resistance.

Those who have diabetes are vulnerable to many threats, including the threat of dehydration. The threat of dehydration is severe and exists daily. This is because when glucose levels increase in the blood, it stimulates the kidneys to increase their function and filter out the excess sugar, resulting in sugar being flushed out of the system via urine. High blood sugar is also concerning because it may lead to the body drawing fluids from important tissues. These could be the lenses of the eyes, brain tissue, and muscle tissue.

Experts always highlight the need to treat dehydration immediately and avoid daily dehydration. This is because it can affect an individual's blood glucose levels. If the body lacks fluids, it leads to the release of a hormone called vasopressin as discussed above. Since it makes the kidneys retain more fluid, the body stores unwanted glucose as those liquids are hoarded. Adding to the concern is that the high levels of vasopressin in the bloodstream stimulate the liver to produce additional blood sugar. The net result of all these factors combined is that it causes insulin resistance. This may also lead to chronic hyperglycemia.

Treatment of dehydration

Dehydration is easy to treat. It is a health problem that can be overcome fast in the cheapest ways. All you need to do is drink more water to overcome this issue. Though experts recommend a minimum amount of water daily, the rules are more complex. This is because the amount of water an individual needs varies and depends on several factors. These are gender, stress levels, physical activity performed, and others. After consulting your doctor, the best course of action is to decide how much water your body needs.

DVT: An Overview

DVT is a blood clot known as deep vein thrombosis. It occurs following a blood clot (thrombus) forming in one or more deep veins. Most commonly, it occurs in the legs. This condition may cause pain in the legs or even swelling. However, at times, individuals may not suffer from any significant symptoms.

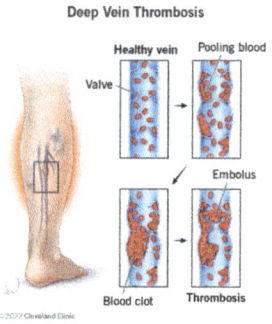

Individuals may suffer from DVT if they have underlying medical conditions that impact the way the blood clots. A blood clot may also form in the legs if the individual has no physical movement for a very long period. Such an instance becomes possible if you only move for a short time, like when traveling long distances or putting on bed rest due to an injury, surgery, or illness.

When DVT and pulmonary embolism combine

Deep vein thrombosis poses considerable risk as the blood clots in the veins can break loose and travel through the bloodstream. They may end up being stuck in the lungs, resulting in blocked blood flow, known as pulmonary embolism, as discussed earlier. However, when DVT and pulmonary embolism occur together, it is known as venous thromboembolism (VTE).

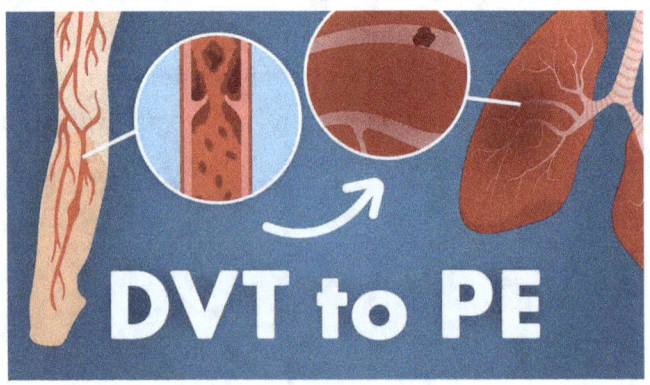

Symptoms and causes of DVT

The symptoms of deep vein thrombosis are leg swelling, pain in the legs, cramping, soreness, skin color changes on the leg, and warmth on the leg. There is also a likelihood that deep vein thrombosis may occur without noticeable symptoms.

The leading cause of deep vein thrombosis is the damage suffered by a vein. This may occur following surgery or inflammation. An infection or injury may also cause the damage.

Risk factors for DVT

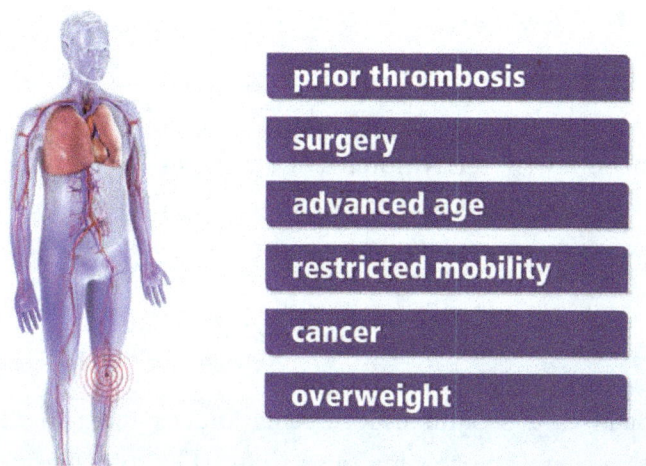

Many factors can increase the risk of developing DVT. Being aged and over 60 increases the risk. However, DVT can also occur at a younger age. Lack of movement is another factor when the legs do not move for a considerable time. The risk is increased when the calf muscles do not contract. Muscle contraction is crucial as it assists in blood flow. Sitting in one place for a long time, such as when traveling long distances in a car, airplane, bus or train further, increase the risks of developing DVT. Long-term bed rest is also another factor. An injury or surgery also increases the risk of blood clots.

Another factor is pregnancy. During pregnancy, pressure in the veins in the pelvis and leg region increases. The risk is also present even six months after the baby has been born. Obese and overweight individuals are also at an increased risk. Those who take birth control pills or undergo hormone replacement therapy also face the threat of DVT.

Smoking impacts blood flow and clots. Some forms of cancers cause an increase in the substances in the bloodstream, causing the blood to clot.

Heart failure makes an individual prone to DVT and pulmonary embolism. Since the heart and lungs in such patients do not function work well, the symptoms of even a small pulmonary embolism may become more aggravated.

Protein C, a natural anticoagulant

Protein C is a naturally occurring anticoagulant in the blood. It helps control the clotting mechanism. The role of anticoagulant is very important as it prevents the blood from clotting. Individuals with a deficiency in Protein C are at an increased risk since they lack the substance (protein C) required to protect the body from excessive clotting.

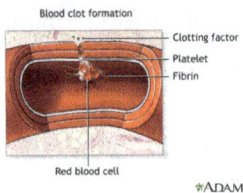

Role of protein C and protein S in preventing blood clotting

Both these proteins in the blood work together to prevent blood clotting mechanisms. Protein C and tests can be conducted to determine how much of these two proteins are in the blood. The test will also help determine how effectively these proteins are performing.

These tests will also help diagnose the inappropriate blood clot in DVT/PE.

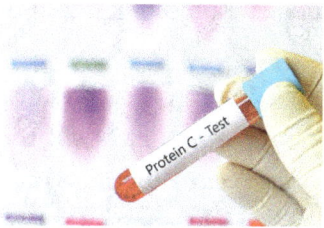

Protein C and S are natural anticoagulants. Studies conducted on these proteins and the subsequent image results show that these proteins are natural anticoagulants.

The body suffers and undergoes a change in the normal balance between clotting and bleeding in case any one of these natural anticoagulants are deficient.

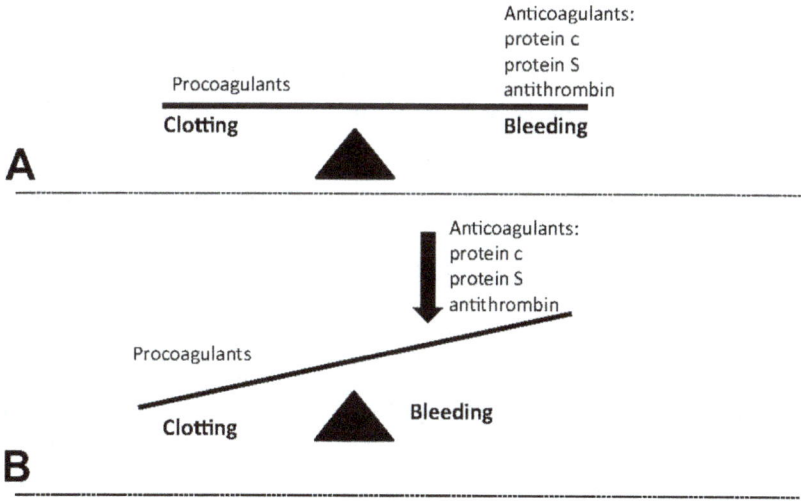

Experts classify the protein C and protein S as glycoproteins synthesized in the liver. They are vital part of the natural anticoagulant system in the body. Both depend on Vitamin K. They are important factors in ensuring adequate physiologic hemostasis maintenance.

A deficiency of protein C and protein S results in the body losing its natural anticoagulant properties. This will then lead to unchecked thrombin generation and eventually cause thromboembolism.

Natural blood thinners in foods

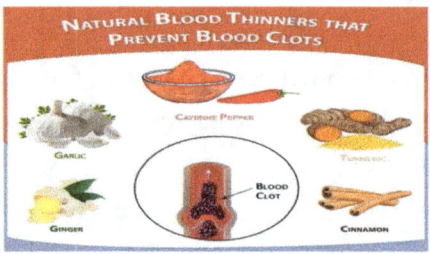

Natural blood thinners are substances found in food. They are helpful for the human body as they reduce the blood's ability to form clots. Though blood clotting is a process required by the body, it can sometimes be dangerous and cause complications if the blood is clotting too much. It can also be potentially dangerous. Hence, such medical issues need to be treated urgently.

Individuals who face certain medical conditions need blood thinning medications. An example is congenital heart defects. Medications in such cases are required to eliminate or reduce the risk of stroke or heart attack.

Some foods serve as natural blood thinners. They help reduce the risk of blood clots. Examples are garlic, ginger, turmeric, beetroot, ginkgo biloba, leafy green vegetables, willow bark, and high-salicylate foods.

It is important to note that not only does having blood that clots easily pose an issue, and having blood that does not clot enough can be a problem. Blood that fails to clot can cause excessive bleeding and anemia.

CHAPTER SEVEN:
DIALYSATE TEMPERATURE AND PH BALANCE

Cooling dialysate - the benefits

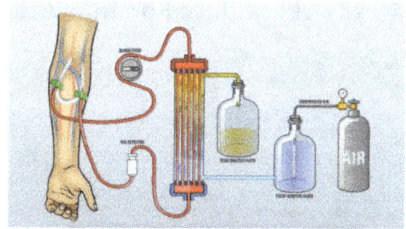

Cooling dialysate traces its history back to when it was utilized as a technique to instill and bring about peripheral vasoconstriction in dialysis. It was also meant to ensure a reduction in intradialytic hypotension incidences. Studies and research have indicated cool dialysate as a potential maneuver to control and prevent intra-dialytic hypotensive (IDH) episodes.

Though only a few studies have thoroughly analyzed of cooled dialysate, the available data points towards improvement in hemodynamic tolerability of dialysis and a protective effect over major organs on employing his technique. The data also confirms that cold dialysis brings about a reduction in cardiovascular mortality and ensures improvement in patients' levels of post-dialysis fatigue. This significantly boosts general health and ensures improved quality of life.

There is considerable evidence to suggest that cold dialysis, through lowering the body core temperature, improves systemic vascular resistance and enhances hemodynamic stability. There are other benefits as well that include avoidance of heat accumulation that brings about counterproductive thermoregulatory vasodilation and ensuring catecholamine surge. The latter is responsible for stimulating peripheral vasoconstriction and cardiac inotropy.

There have been proven benefits of long-term cold dialysis. These benefits occur in both brain and heart tissues. Cold dialysis incites a positive change in the brain region by inducing a protective effect from injurious perfusion of the cerebral vascular beds. It does so by reducing the impact of HD- induced brain injuries.

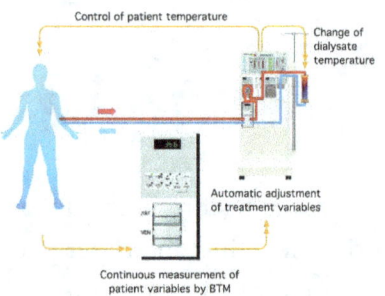

There are obvious benefits for the heart as well. Carrying out long-term induction of cold dialysis incites positive changes in resting ejection fraction. Also, there were significant reductions in both left ventricular mass and end-diastolic volumes. Overall, it served to minimize the risks of sustaining cardiovascular issues in the future.

Studies suggest cold dialysis does not incur changes in blood volume, urea rebound, or effective Kt/V index. However, some studies indicate significant improvements in urea removal and Kt/V.

The benefits of cooler dialysate solution at a glance:

Here are some of the benefits measured by employing a cooler dialysate solution:

- Reduce incidences of intradialytic hypotension
- Ensures hemodynamic stability
- Reduction in ischemic brain injuries
- Helping preserve the brain's white matter
- Improvement in cardiac functionality
- Controlling arterial blood pressure when performing hemodialysis
- Reduction witnessed in post-dialysis fatigue
- Boost energy levels
- Dialysis efficiency remains unchanged
- Undergoing improvement in the overall health
- Leading to a decrease in the times nursing intervention is required during HD

How is cold dialysis achieved?

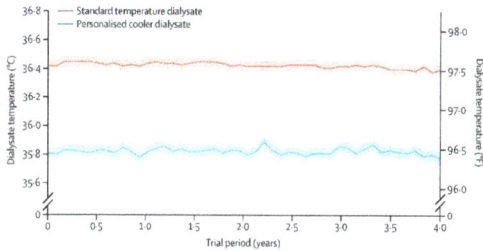

To achieve this purpose, the dialysate temperature must be cooled to 35 °C-36 °C or 0.5 °C below resting body temperature. No additional costs are required to implement cold dialysis, and this method is universally applicable. Though cooling the dialysate solution reduces intradialytic hypotension incidences and even increases energy levels, it could also discomfort the patients.

Importance of maintaining the body's pH levels

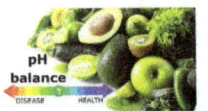

Water is the basic need of all living organisms. It has a neutral pH level of 7.0. The ideal pH for a human body is between 7.30 and 7.45. The pH is a measure of hydrogen ion concentration. If the pH turns acidic by dropping below the ideal optimum pH, it could affect the organs and tissues. One possible consequence of an acidic pH inside the body is that it can lead to acid reflux, heartburn, or inflammation in the digestive organ. Also, an acidic body is the ideal breeding ground for pathogens.

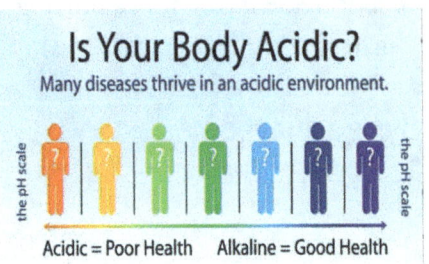

Acid reflux: An overview

Acid reflux occurs when the body's pH level becomes acidic, and some of it flows from the stomach into the esophagus. Heartburn refers to a burning sensation an individual feels following an acid reflux. If there are frequent cases of acid reflux, then it may cause the person to suffer from GERD. Heartburn is classified as a symptom of acid reflux. It is important to note that heartburn is not associated with the heart in any way.

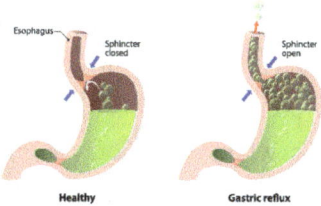

On the other hand, gastroesophageal reflux disease (GERD) is a severe form of the disease that the doctor diagnoses if an individual is undergoing acid reflux frequently. It usually happens if there is an acid reflux twice every week.

GERD is a common condition in western countries that affects an estimated 20% of the total population in the Western hemisphere. Around 20% of Americans are afflicted with this condition when speaking about the U.S. alone.

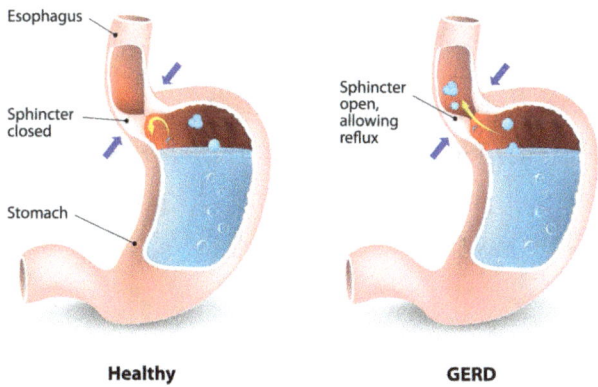

Atherosclerosis and its Connection with Acidity

Too much acid causes the blood vessels to line themselves with fatty plaques called Atherosclerosis. However, before delving into details about Atherosclerosis, it is important to distinguish between Atherosclerosis and Arteriosclerosis. This is because though they refer to the same condition yet, there is a difference between these two terms. Arteriosclerosis is when the blood vessels carrying oxygen and nutrients become thick and stiff. These vessels also carry nutrients from the heart to other body parts. This restricts the blood flow to the tissues and organs.

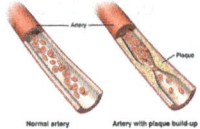

Though healthy arteries have the features of being elastic and flexible, the walls in the arteries can harden, which leads to the hardening of the arteries.

On the other hand, Atherosclerosis is a specific type of arteriosclerosis and refers to the buildup of fats and cholesterol on the artery walls. They may also accumulate inside the artery wall, a condition known as plaque. The plaque leads to the narrowing of the arteries, thereby inhibiting blood flow. At times, the plaque may also burst, resulting in blood clots.

Atherosclerosis is not just a heart problem

There is a common misconception that Atherosclerosis may be a heart problem. However, Atherosclerosis can impact arteries in any part of the body. The good news is that Atherosclerosis can be treated, and living a healthy lifestyle prevents this condition from occurring.

Atherosclerosis and mesenteric ischemia

Atherosclerosis causes the arteries responsible for supplying blood to the intestines to narrow down. This may lead to mesenteric ischemia. In this condition, an individual feels belly pain after eating. It occurs because the body attempts to increase blood supply to the gut but fails to do so.

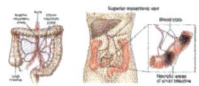

Atherosclerosis and Ischemic strokes

When acid causes the blood vessels to line themselves with fatty plaques (atherosclerosis), it leads to the formation of blood clots blocking blood flow and hence oxygen to the brain. This is known as Ischemic strokes. This situation can contribute to cardiovascular disease.

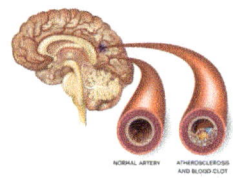

This is not the only condition endured by the body due to atherosclerosis occurring in the arteries that lead to the brain. The person may feel numbness and weakness in the legs and arms, followed by difficulty speaking (slurred speech). At times, it may result in temporary vision loss in one eye. This is a precursor to a transient ischemic attack (TIA). If left untreated, this condition may lead to a stroke. If atherosclerosis occurs in the heart arteries, it may lead to chest pain, known as angina.

How is the plaque formed?

Inflammation and other factors, such as obesity, age, diabetes, insulin resistance, high blood pressure, and high cholesterol, may cause damage to the inner wall of an artery. Blood vessels and other substances may accumulate on the injury site, leading to a buildup on the artery's inner lining. As time passes, the fats and cholesterol may accumulate on the heart arteries' inner walls, leading to a buildup known as plaque. Plaque is a serious condition as it causes the arteries to narrow down, blocking blood flow. The plaque may also burst at times, resulting in a blood clot.

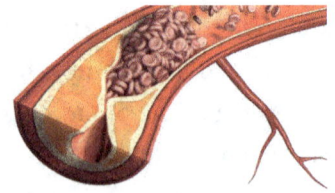

Atherosclerosis may also be caused by high C-reactive protein (CRP) levels. This is because CRP is also a marker of inflammation. Other possible causes include lack of exercise, sleep apnea, and smoking.

Possible complications

The complications will depend on the type of arteries that have been blocked or narrowed down due to atherosclerosis.

If Atherosclerosis causes the arteries near your heart to narrow down, this leads to coronary heart disease. This may lead to angina or a heart attack.

Suppose the arteries leading to the brain are narrowed down. In that case, it may cause carotid artery disease, which can lead to a transient ischemic attack (TIA) and even a stroke in the future, as mentioned earlier.

If atherosclerosis occurs in the arteries leading to your arms and legs, it may lead to peripheral artery disease. Blood flow problems in the arms and legs mark this condition. This condition leads to the body becoming less sensitive to heat and cold. This increases the risks of burns and frostbite. In rare conditions, the condition may turn grave, causing tissue death, known as gangrene.

Aneurysms are another condition caused by atherosclerosis. This serious condition that may occur in any part of the body. However, the dangerous part is that it usually has no symptoms. It may result in pain in areas afflicted by aneurysms, leading to a medical emergency. In some cases, the aneurysms may burst, causing life-threatening bleeding inside the body.

If the arteries leading to the kidneys narrow down, it will prevent the blood cells rich in oxygen from reaching the kidneys, resulting in chronic kidney disease. It is important to mention that the kidneys require sufficient blood to filter waste products and remove excess fluid.

Preventing atherosclerosis

Healthy lifestyle changes can prevent atherosclerosis. These are the lifestyle changes required to keep the arteries healthy. They are:

- Intake of healthy foods
- Quitting tobacco (both smoking and smokeless tobacco)
- Regular exercises
- Maintaining a healthy weight
- Maintaining healthy BP
- Maintaining healthy cholesterol levels
- Maintaining healthy blood sugar levels

The connection between gout and uric acid

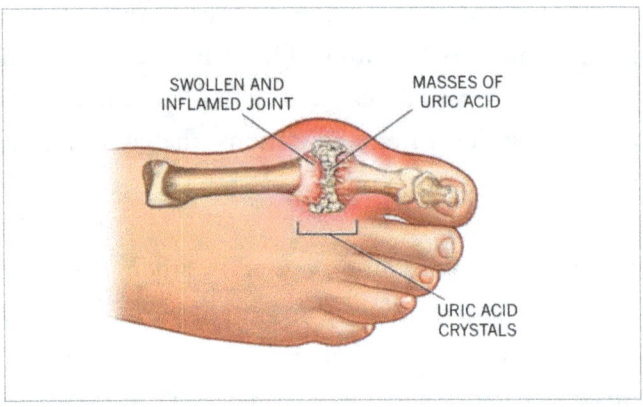

Excess acid or deposits of uric acid crystals may accumulate in the joints due to high blood levels of uric acid (hyperuricemia), leading to a disorder known as gout. When these uric acid crystals accumulate in the joints, they may cause painful inflammation known as flares (attacks). This may also affect movement and cause undesired pain.

Gout (Inflamatory Arthritis)

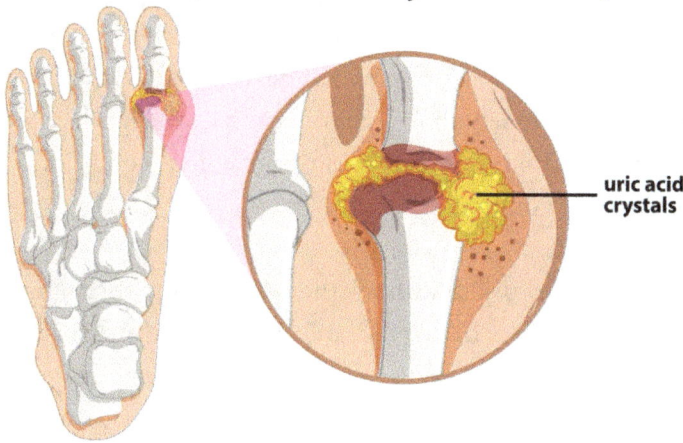

When uric acid crystals accumulate in the joint, the inflamed joint is diagnosed as gout after fluid removed from the affected joint shows uric crystal acids. This condition is treated with medication that decreases inflammation and relieves pain. In most cases, the patients may need to take medications for a lifetime. They need these medications to decrease blood levels of uric acid.

How is uric acid formed?

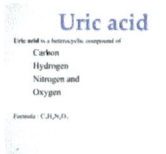

Uric acid is created as a by-product of the breakdown of nucleic acids (ribonucleic acid) and deoxyribonucleic acid (DNA). This breakdown occurs in the cells. Even under normal conditions, uric acid is present in the body in small amounts in the blood because the cells undergo continuous breakdown, with new cells forming. The body is also responsible for transforming foods, purines, into uric acid. These purines are the building blocks of RNA and DNA.

Causes of gout

Gout is more common among males than females. Developing most commonly in middle-aged men, it develops after menopause in women. As mentioned above, gout is caused by high levels of uric acid in the blood, known as hyperuricemia. This condition is often found to run in families.

The body removes uric acid from the body mainly through the kidneys. The gastrointestinal system also removes some uric acid. High uric acid levels in the blood may occur due to some reasons. Most importantly, high levels result from the kidneys and gastrointestinal system eliminating less uric acid. When the kidneys cannot eliminate enough uric acid through urine, the uric acid levels in the blood become abnormally higher. This may occur even if the kidney function is normal and result from genes. This means that the uric acid in the blood forms uric acid crystals and deposits in or around the joints.

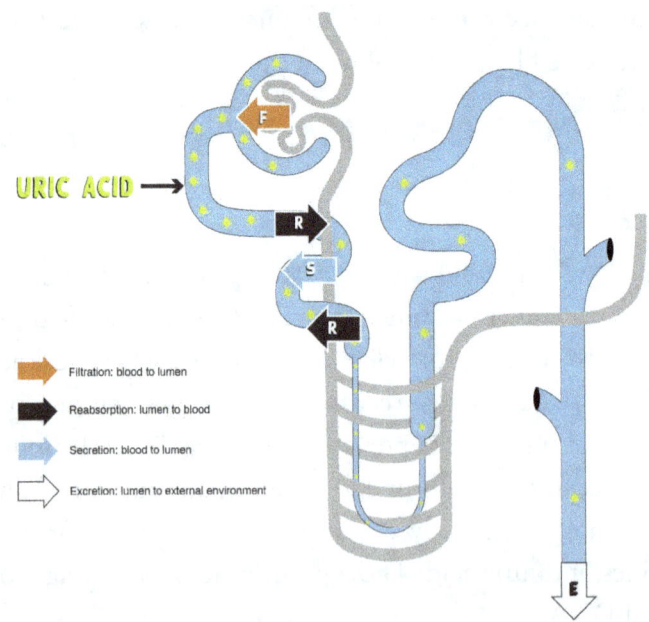

In other cases, conditions may impair the kidney's functioning and affect its ability to remove uric acids, such as some types of kidney diseases, certain drugs, and lead poisoning.

Consuming too much purine-rich food can also cause the problem. Such food includes red meat, shellfish, kidney, asparagus, herring, mushrooms, mussels, sardines, and meat gravies. These foods can increase the uric acid level in the blood. Though it may be essential to suggest that such foods cause uric acid crystals, it must also be noted that following a low-purine diet only lowers uric acid levels by an insignificant amount. Such therapy may not be the solution if an individual is diagnosed with gout.

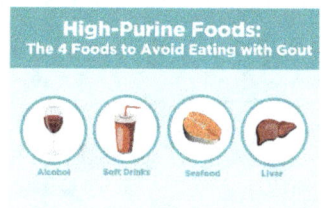

Still, it is vital to avoid an intake of a high-purine diet with too much alcohol. It must also not be combined with beverages that contain high-fructose corn syrup. Such beverages cause a rise in uric acid production and cause problems for the kidneys eliminating uric acid.

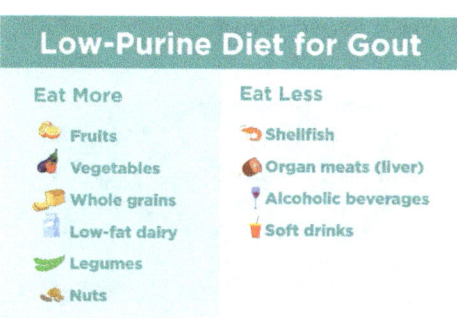

At times, acute gouty arthritis may form without any warnings. This may occur due to an injury, surgery, illness, certain medications, and consumption of purine-rich foods and alcohol.

Cancer and malignant cells

Cancer refers to the abnormal growth of cells. These cells multiply in an acidic environment and eventually die. However, some of dead cells adapt and find a way to thrive by undergoing changes and becoming malignant. These malignant cells are not normal cells formed due to the DNA memory code in humans. These cells are derived from a single abnormal cell. The different part about these cells is that they have undergone changes causing them to lose standard control mechanisms.

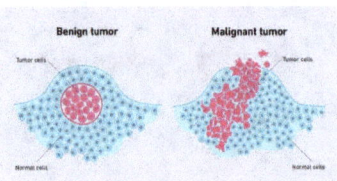

The cancer cells can multiply continuously, usually invading nearby tissues, and may even move to other parts of the body. Following such a migration, they promote new blood vessel growth and derive nutrients from these sources. These cancerous or malignant cells may develop in any tissue of the body.

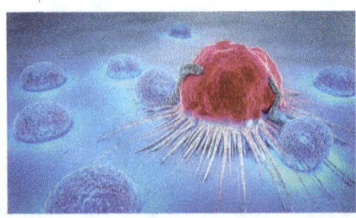

With the cancerous cells growing and multiplying, a mass of cancerous tissue, known as a tumor, is formed. This then leads to the normal adjacent tissues being invaded and destroyed. A Tumor is a medical term used to describe abnormal growth or mass. These tumors may be cancerous or noncancerous. The different part about cancerous cells is that they may spread from the initial source to other parts of the body in a process known as metastasizing.

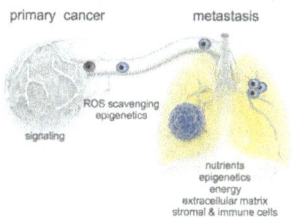

Production of acid by cancer cells

Once the cancer cells grow, they produce more acid, making it difficult for the body to raise pH levels. Since toxins are acidic, the blood needs to have neutral pH.

Intake of a low-acid diet helps fight cancer by controlling inflammation in the body.

Hence, with lots of fluids, an alkaline diet of fruits and vegetables, such as apples, blueberries, lemons, grapes, soybeans, almonds, wild rice, green tea, etc., will help the cause.

It is important to avoid acidic foods, like carbonated beverages and energy drinks, popcorn, cheese and cream cheese, pork and red meats, beer and wine, pasta, oats, white bread, pastries, sweetened fruit juices, wheat, peanut, nuts and roasted nuts, soy milk, barley, and black tea.

Cancer metabolism and control by cutting off glucose supply

Cancer metabolism thrives when the cancer cells ensure their survival through a process known as symbiosis. In this process, one cancer cell starts producing lactate with ATP production. For this purpose, glucose is consumed, while the neighboring cancer cell starts consuming the secreted lactate, producing ATP. The ATP is produced via the TCA cycle and oxidative phosphorylation.

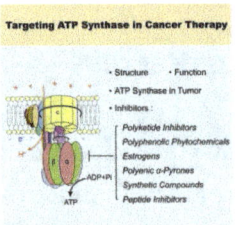

Since the cancer cells usually depend on glycolysis primarily to produce ATP, controlling ATP is important. The cancer cells need to consume more fuel, such as glucose, to produce ATP for survival. Hence, the patient should not be given sugars. This will block the lactic acid, allowing the cancer cells to generate ATP and improving the immune system's ability to destroy the abnormal cells that utilize phagocytosis.

CHAPTER EIGHT:
STROKE AND HTN

The connection between High Salt Diet, Stroke and HTN

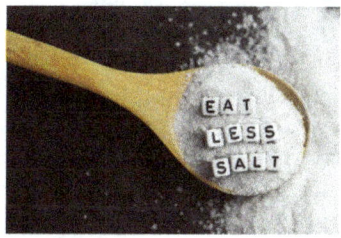

Blood pressure and kidneys have an important connection. When the bean-shaped organs are damaged or injured, the heart and blood pressure are at the receiving end.

Kidneys are responsible for filtering more than 120 quarts of blood daily. The kidneys excrete toxins and unwanted fluid from the body's cells and send them to the bladder to be excreted via urine.

The problem with a high salt intake is that it makes it harder for the kidneys to remove the unwanted fluid. The result is that the fluid builds up in the system, causing the blood pressure to increase.

Salt intake and impact on the heart

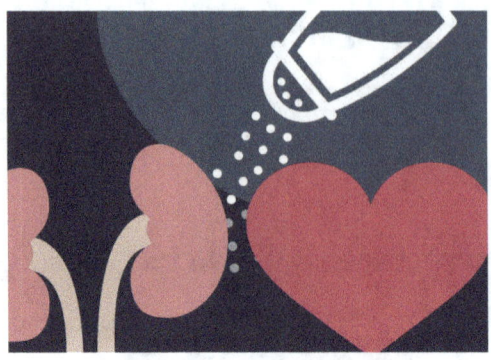

Intake of excessive salt over time leads to high blood pressure, also known as Hypertension. This condition causes the blood vessels to stiffen and narrow, decreasing blood and oxygen to the body's key organs. This development forces the heart to pump harder to ensure blood flows throughout the body. This leads to a further increase in blood pressure. High blood pressure has consequences, especially if it persists for a long time, as it puts enormous strain on the heart. It causes the heart's left pumping chamber to enlarge, weakening the heart muscle and eventually causing heart failure.

Hypertension, if left unchecked, damages the artery walls. The artery walls start collecting fat, which leads to heart disease and possibly results in a heart attack or stroke. Experts often cite that the best and most effective way to prevent a heart attack is to ensure the arteries are not damaged.

Impact of hypertension on the Kidneys

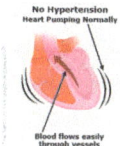
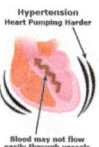

The impact of high salt intake described in the above section often spells kidney trouble, resulting in kidney disease. Hypertension results in extra pressure on the kidneys' filtering units, causing scarring. This development impairs the kidneys' function. Its ability to regulate fluid is affected, leading to increased blood pressure.

If this cycle continues unchecked, the possible outcomes are kidney disease and kidney failure.

The two most important reasons for kidney disease are high blood pressure and uncontrolled diabetes.

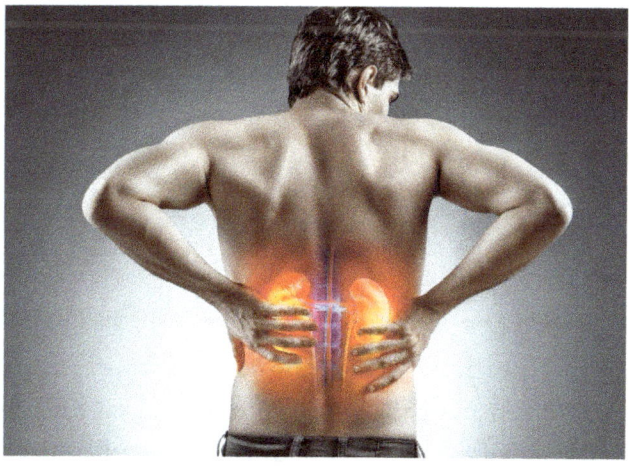

The sad part is that most of those with kidney disease fail to realize the gravity of the situation. The signs and symptoms visible initially may be mistaken for other conditions or may become apparent once the kidneys have started to fail. To avoid this complication, here are the symptoms to look out for:

- Fatigue
- Difficulty sleeping
- Itchy skin
- Decrease in urination
- Blood in the urine
- Swelling in the feet or ankles
- Swelling around the eyes
- Drop in appetite
- Nausea
- Vomiting
- Muscle cramps
- Confusion in mental status
- Abnormal taste

Suppose symptoms are present and especially if you are aged above 60 and have high blood pressure or diabetes with a family history of kidney failure. In that case, you need to see a kidney expert immediately.

How salt affects people

Salt has a different effect on people, with some being able to consume sodium without affecting their blood pressure. However, people who are 'salt sensitive' may harm their kidneys even with a slight sodium increase. It would affect their kidneys' ability to regulate fluid, increasing blood pressure.

Salt sensitivity is common among elderly and middle-aged individuals. It is also common among those who are obese or black. Its intensity increases as an individual ages.

Lifestyle changes matter a lot

Modifying your lifestyle helps the cause. This can be ensured in the following ways:

- Intake of a low-sodium diet
- Avoiding alcohol
- Regular exercises
- Maintaining a healthy weight.

However, it is important to note that blood pressure may remain elevated despite restricting salt intake and following healthy lifestyle changes. In such cases, medications would be required apart from the above lifestyle changes to reduce blood pressure. Examples of such medications are mentioned below:

- Diuretics or water pills (These will increase urination and help eliminate the excess fluid)
- Angiotensin-converting enzyme (ACE) inhibitors (to relax blood vessels)
- Angiotensin II receptor blockers (ARBs) (to relax blood vessels)

Apart from keeping hypertension and diabetes in check, yearly testing for kidney disease is recommended.

One way to ensure the health and longevity of the heart and kidneys is to consult a doctor to ensure the salt intake does not increase your blood pressure and, thereby, does not impact the heart and kidneys.

The most common sources of sodium

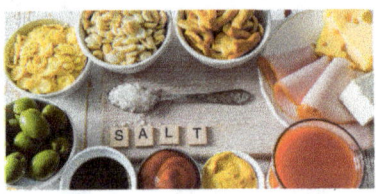

Most Americans have a great liking for a high-salt diet. Skipping table salt is a meaningful way to cut the salt intake. The problem is that most of the sodium in the diet comes in the shape of processed or packaged foods. Reducing the consumption of such foods reduces sodium intake and helps lower blood pressure. It is an essential step in preventing hypertension.

The American Heart Association's recommendation

The American Heart Association has recommended keeping the salt intake lower than 2,300 mgs. The ideal limit is no more than 1,500 mg daily, especially if the individual has high blood pressure. Studies have shown that cutting salt intake by 1,000 mg a day helps improve blood pressure and enhances overall heart health.

Here are some substances that increase the risk of Hypertension:

- Processed foods
- Natural foods containing high sodium content (seafood, cheese, olives)
- Table salt
- Sea salt
- Kosher salt

- Some OTC drugs
- Certain prescription medications

A brief overview: How does salt impact the balance of sodium concentration in the blood

Here is more on the impact of salt on the blood pressure. Salt consists of 40% sodium and 60% chloride. Sodium is vital for the body as it is required to balance water and minerals. It is also necessary to conduct nerve impulses and ensure smooth contraction and relaxation of the muscles. Consuming excess salt means that the body needs to hold on to more water to balance the blood's sodium concentration. This leads to an increased amount of water in the body, resulting in increased blood volume.

Since more blood is made to flow through the arteries, the blood pressure increases. The problem is that, in the long run, the increased pressure on the arteries may cause them to either narrow down or harden. This leads to plaque buildup, which then blocks the blood vessels. The net result of the extra water in the body is bloating and an imbalance in body fluid homeostasis.

The impact described above may be more vigorous among individuals more sensitive to salt. A few factors, such as weight, age, ethnicity, and any existing medical conditions, can influence salt's effects on the blood pressure.

Other concerning aspects of high salt intake

Salt does not only affect the heart and blood pressure. It causes problems for the entire body. In individuals with high blood pressure, the kidneys are prone to holding on to excess salt instead of the natural response of eliminating the salt. This leads to new health issues, such as swollen ankles. Another primary concern is the buildup of fluid around the heart and lungs. This has been discussed later in this chapter.

Excess salt also has the potential to harm the brain by damaging arteries and increasing blood pressure. This may lead to an increase in the risk of stroke and dementia. It may also end up harming the brain stem. The Brain stem is an important function as it regulates blood pressure and salt balance.

Studies have also shown that salt may affect the immune system. It is also a precursor to inflammation, contributing to heart disease and other health issues. The inflammation and high BP are caused by the salt's effect on gut bacteria.

Hemorrhagic Stroke: An Overview

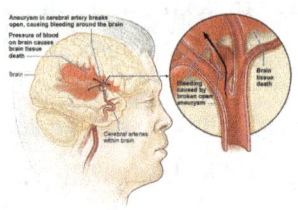

A hemorrhagic stroke results from blood from an artery suddenly bleeding in the brain. This means that the damaged brain part causes the part of the body under its control to stop working correctly.

Hemorrhagic stroke has been classified into two types. The first type is intracranial hemorrhages where the bleeding happens inside the brain. The second is subarachnoid hemorrhages, where bleeding occurs between the brain and its membranes.

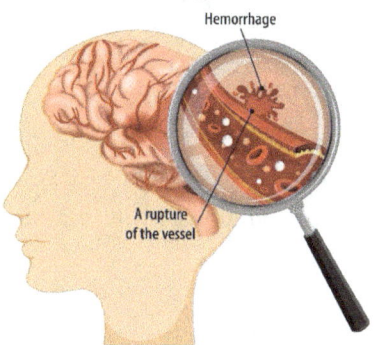

Symptoms of hemorrhagic stroke

The possible symptoms of a stroke warrant urgent medical attention. The outcome is better the sooner medical treatment is offered as only a few brain cells would be damaged in this case.

There are some signs of stroke, such as:

- Sudden confusion in mental state
- Sudden numbness occurring in the arm, face, or leg. This
- occurs especially in only one side of the body
- Sudden difficulty in seeing with one or both the eyes
- Difficulty in walking
- Sudden dizziness
- Loss of coordination
- Severe headache that has a sudden onset
- Difficulty speaking

There are additional symptoms as well:

- One side of the body becomes paralyzed
- Body becomes sensitive to light
- Stiffness occurs in the neck, resulting in neck pain\
- Frequent fluctuations occur in the heartbeat
- Fluctuations in breathing
- Hand tremors are felt
- Difficulty faced in swallowing
- Feeling of an abnormal taste in the mouth

Causes of hemorrhagic stroke

As mentioned above, hemorrhagic stroke may result from sudden bleeding from a blood vessel inside the brain. The sudden bleeding may be the result of a head injury, high BP, cerebral aneurysm, arteriovenous malformation (AVM) or amyloid angiopathy, brain disease, drug abuse, a blood disorder, liver disease, bleeding disorders (an example is sickle cell anemia),

How HTN leads to heart attack

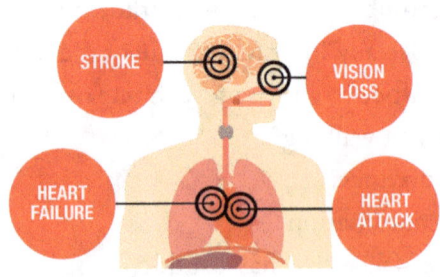

An excess strain is caused by high blood pressure causing damage to the artery. The coronary arteries leading to the heart start narrowing as plaque forms, which is an accumulation of fat and cholesterol mostly (may contain other substances) in a slow process known as atherosclerosis (mentioned in Chapter 7).

Once the arteries harden due plaque, blood clots will likely form. Once an artery is blocked due to plaque or a blood clot, the blood flow through the heart muscle becomes affected. This interruption starves the heart muscle of oxygen and nutrients. This results in damage or death of the affected part of the heart muscle, leading to a heart attack.

Fluid buildup around the heart and lungs due to HTN

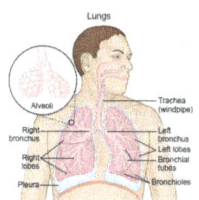

Pulmonary edema is a medical condition resulting from too much fluid accumulation in the lungs. This fluid accumulates in the air sacs that are found in the lungs. This condition makes it difficult for an individual to breathe.

Most commonly, pulmonary edema is caused by heart problems. However, there are other reasons why fluid may collect in the lungs. Such causes include pneumonia, medications, chest wall trauma, and exercising at high elevations. Coming in contact with certain toxins is another reason.

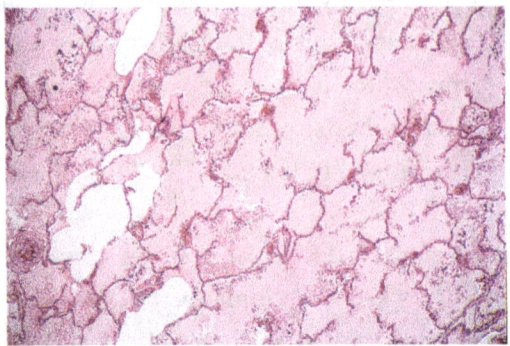

Pulmonary edema may also develop suddenly and is known as acute pulmonary edema. This condition requires urgent medical attention. Pulmonary edema is a dangerous condition and may, at times, also cause death. However, receiving prompt medical treatment will help alleviate the condition. The pulmonary edema treatment depends on the cause. However, it commonly includes oxygen and medications.

Since pulmonary edema is caused by an abnormal fluid buildup in the lungs, it can cause shortness of breath.

Causes of pulmonary edema

This condition most commonly occurs due to congestive heart failure. Once the heart fails to pump blood efficiently, blood may flow back into the veins responsible for taking blood through the lungs.

The fluid gets pushed into the air spaces after the pressure increases in these blood vessels. The air spaces are found in the lungs and are known as alveoli. This fluid then causes the normal oxygen movement to be affected. Both these factors together result in shortness of breath.

Suppose the pulmonary edema is caused by congestive heart failure. In that case, it may be due to a heart attack or a heart disease that causes the heart muscle to stiffen or weaken, also known as cardiomyopathy. The narrowed heart valves, the mitral or aortic valves, may also cause it. Sudden hypertension may also be the cause.

There are other reasons for causing pulmonary edema, such as certain medications, exposure to high altitude, arteries bringing blood to kidneys narrowing down, kidney failure, lung damage due to poisonous gas or severe infection ,and a significant injury.

Salt and its connection with CA homeostasis and Osteoporosis

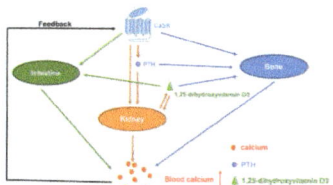

Salt has been identified as the reason behind the increase in the urinary excretion of calcium. This is the reason why it is considered a high-risk factor for osteoporosis. This increase in the urinary excretion of calcium owing to a higher sodium intake can be addressed if the intestinal system ensures increased absorption of dietary calcium.

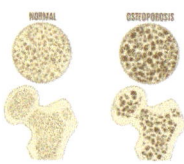

Diets that are a possible risk factor include ones with a high sodium content that potentially alter calcium metabolism through an increase in urinary calcium excretion, known as calcinuria (calcium salts found in the urine). Hence, a diet with a high salt intake increases the risk of osteoporosis.

Calcium homeostasis is an important process managed by the hormones regulating calcium transport in different body parts, such as gut, bone and kidneys. There are three primary hormones responsible for this task. They are:

- Parathyroid hormone (PTH)
- 1,25-dihydroxy vitamin D-3 (Vitamin D3)
- calcitonin

Role of salt in controlling the amount of calcium in the urine

Salt plays a major role in controlling the amount of calcium in the urine. It also controls the amount of calcium lost from the bones. Since calcium is necessary for maintaining bone strength, an increased salt intake weakens bones and hence causes osteoporosis.

In chronic Dialysis Patients, the ability to urinate is affected, which then causes calcification, which means the calcium deposits onto the arteries/tissues, causing them to harden.

Calcification

This process refers to calcium buildup in body tissue, which hardens tissue. However, this process may either be normal or abnormal.

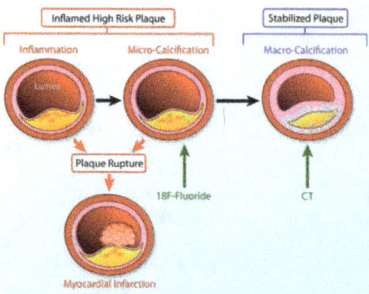

A massive chunk of calcium (almost 99%) is deposited on the bones and teeth in the body. The remaining 1% of calcium gets dissolved in the blood.

What happens when the balance between calcium and certain chemicals is affected?

If a disorder results in the balance between calcium and certain chemicals in the body being upset, the calcium, and in other parts of the body. These could be the arteries, brain, kidneys and lungs. Calcium deposits are problematic as they affect how these blood vessels and organs function. Calcifications are usually visible on X-rays. An example of this condition is calcium deposits occurring in the arteries. This is a part of atherosclerosis.

Role of Alkalinizers in reducing inflammation

Green leafy vegetables, also known as Alkalinizers, are good sources of dietary nutrients and potassium. These can help the body improve blood vessel function and reduce inflammation, preventing the process that leads to Arteriosclerosis.

CHAPTER NINE:
LAB VALUES INVOLVED IN DIALYSIS AND ASSESSMENT PROCESS

Hemodialysis: An Overview

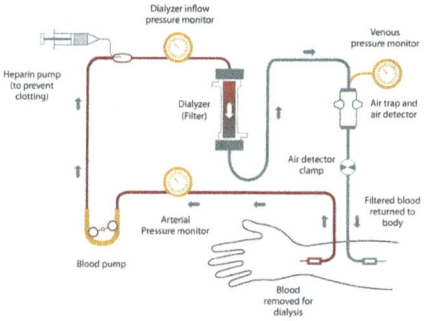

Hemodialysis is when a machine filters wastes, salts, and fluid in the bloodstream. Staying on hemodialysis becomes mandatory in case the kidneys are unhealthy to perform this function properly. This is an advanced form of treatment that treats kidney failure. With hemodialysis, a person with kidney failure can continue to live an active and healthy life.

Hemodialysis as an important responsibility

Hemodialysis needs to be conducted regularly, and the process must be flawless. Patients must follow a few fundamental principles closely to make their treatment more effective. Starting with medications, they need to be taken regularly and on time-however, the entire responsibility is not only on the patient. A healthcare team works closely with the patient to ensure hemodialysis is a success. This team includes a kidney doctor, nurse, and other healthcare professionals skilled and experienced at managing such cases. Hemodialysis can also be conducted at home.

When does hemodialysis become necessary

Hemodialysis becomes necessary if the doctor decides there is no other way out. For this purpose, several factors are taken into consideration before making this decision. These factors include the overall health of the patient, kidney function, the signs and symptoms present, quality of life, and the patient's personal preferences.

Since symptoms of kidney failure are devastating, such as vomiting, swelling, fatigue, and nausea, prompt treatment is necessary. The kidney function is measured through the glomerular filtration rate (eGFR). The eFGR is calculated by performing blood creatinine test results and considering the patient's sex, age, and other factors. The typical value usually varies with age. However, measuring kidney function is extremely important as it helps a doctor plan the treatment procedure.

Hemodialysis is of utmost importance. Even in people with kidney failure, a healthcare team through hemodialysis can manage the patient's blood pressure and ensure adequate maintenance of a proper balance of fluid and various minerals. The fluids include potassium and sodium in the body. It is also important to mention that hemodialysis must be started before your kidneys cease functioning. This is necessary to avoid life-threatening complications.

A brief reminder: Most common causes of kidney failure

As mentioned in the earlier chapters, kidney failure occurs due to certain factors. These include diabetes, hypertension, inherited kidney disease, kidney cysts, and using anti-inflammatory drugs for a long time.

Preparing for hemodialysis

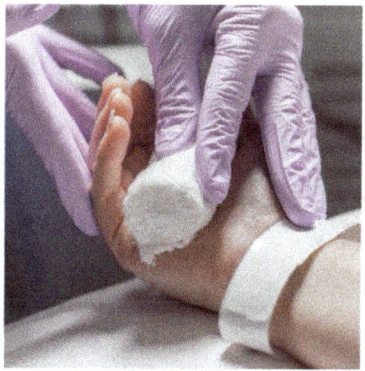

Hemodialysis preparation must commence several weeks or even months before the first procedure is performed on the patient. Starting the procedure requires the surgeon to access your bloodstream easily. For this purpose, vascular access is created that paves the way to create a mechanism to safely remove a small amount of blood from the circulatory system and return it to the patient once it has undergone treatment.

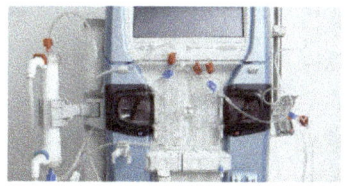

An important guideline that needs to be followed is that surgical access requires time for healing. Healing of the access is necessary for beginning hemodialysis treatment, even though it takes time.

The different types of accesses

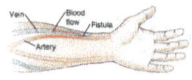

The first type of surgical access is an arteriovenous (AV) fistula. A connection must be made between an artery and a vein to surgically create an AV fistula. This is commonly made on the arm and used less often by the patient. This access is preferred on account of its effectiveness and safety.

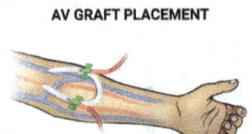

The second type of access is the AV graft. At times, a patient may have blood vessels that are too small, meaning an AV fistula cannot be formed. Hence, the surgeon must choose this method by creating a pathway between an artery and a vein. This is achieved through the use of a tube called a flexible graft.

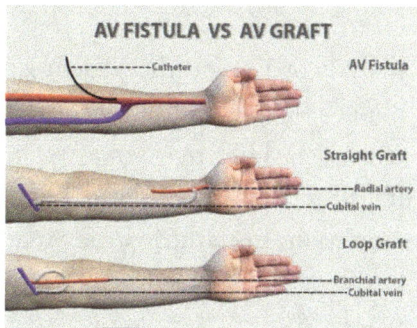

The third type of access is a central venous catheter. This access is usually gained in cases of emergency hemodialysis. In this method, a plastic tube called a catheter is inserted into a large vein in the neck. In such cases, the catheter is only for temporary usage.

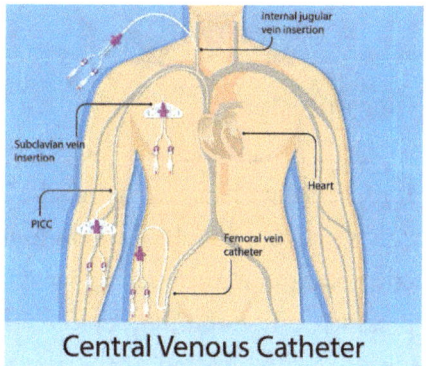

As a nurse, doctor, or any other healthcare professional involved in the hemodialysis process, extreme caution must be exercised to look after the access site. This is because the possibility of infection always looms large. Care is also required to avoid other complications.

The hemodialysis procedure

During the hemodialysis treatment, the patient is made to sit or recline in a chair. Blood is made to flow through the dialyzer. The dialyzer is made to act as a filter that serves as an artificial kidney. Patients are encouraged to wait for TV, read a book, or nap-usually, who receive dialysis at night sleep during the procedure.

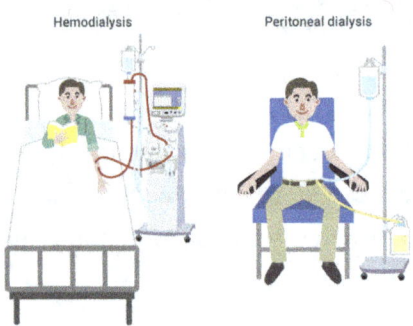

Preparation of the procedure

Before the procedure is initiated and as part of the pre- hemodialysis assessment protocols, the team involved, including the nurse, must take various patient measurements, such as weight and vital signs, including blood pressure, pulse and temperature. The skin needs to be specifically cleansed at the location of the access site from where the blood will leave and then reenter the patient's body.

LAB VALUES INVOLVED IN DIALYSIS AND ASSESSMENT PROCESS 153

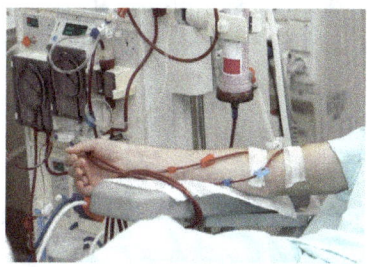

Starting hemodialysis

During the treatment, a surgeon will insert two needles into the patient's arm through the access site. These needles will be taped to remain in place and secure. The two needles will be fixed to a plastic tube connected to a dialyzer. The dialyzer will filter the blood through one tube at the rate of a few ounces each time. This will allow the wastes and extra fluids to leave your bloodstream by passing into a cleansing fluid. This cleansing fluid serves as the dialysate. Once the blood has been filtered, it will be returned to the body through the second tube.

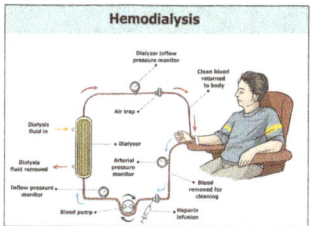

Symptoms during hemodialysis

When hemodialysis is performed, the patient may feel nausea and abdominal cramps. This happens because the excess fluid is withdrawn from the patient's body. The symptoms are more prevalent if the patient accumulates a significant amount of fluid between the dialysis sessions. If the patient feels uncomfortable during hemodialysis, the healthcare professionals must try to alleviate the symptoms through different measures. This may require the need to adjust the speed of hemodialysis. Medications may also need to be adjusted along with the hemodialysis fluids.

Monitoring during hemodialysis

> **Monitoring During Dialysis**
> - Vital Signs
>   - Monitor as per your center
> - Monitor the patients behavior, appearance, response and symptoms
> - Give medications as prescribed
> - Monitor the machine for alarms

The process of hemodialysis requires close monitoring. As a healthcare professional, especially a nurse, blood pressure and heart rate must be monitored and checked often during hemodialysis. There is a need to check the vital signs many times since the blood pressure and heart rate keep fluctuating during the withdrawal of excess fluid.

Finishing part

Once the hemodialysis process has been completed, the needles must be removed from the access site. A pressure dressing must be carefully applied to the access site to avoid bleeding. The patient's weight will need to be re-recorded. After that, the patient is free to engage in activities until the time for the next session starts.

Results and significance

For patients with acute kidney injury, hemodialysis is required for a short time and can be ceased once the kidneys have recovered. However, if the kidney has suffered from reduced kidney function due to a sudden injury, the probability of full recovery is diminished. In such cases, independence from hemodialysis may not be possible.

The hemodialysis team will continue monitoring the patient's treatment to ensure the treatment is on the right track and that the hemodialysis successfully removes enough waste from the blood. Throughout the process and after the treatment, the weight and blood pressure will be monitored closely.

Tests required by hemodialysis patients and their results

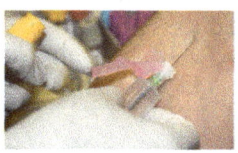

The hemodialysis patient will need to undergo many tests every month. They are discussed below.

- Blood tests to measure urea reduction ratio (URR)
- Total urea clearance (Kt/V) (This will measure how successful is the hemodialysis procedure in removing waste

- Blood chemistry evaluation
- Assessment of blood counts
- Measuring the flow of blood occurring through the access site during the process

The test results will allow the hemodialysis care team to make proper adjustments in the hemodialysis intensity and frequency to benefit the patient.

Some of the most essential tests that are required for a hemodialysis patient are being discussed.

Serum creatinine

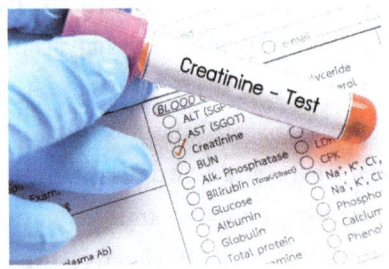

This test aims to determine the amount of creatinine available in the bloodstream. The usual range of this test lies between 0.8 to 1.4 milligrams per deciliter (mg/dl). This test takes a blood sample and sends it for analysis. This test needs to be conducted during the early and later stages of CKD. It must also be conducted during end-stage renal disease (ESRD).

LAB VALUES INVOLVED IN DIALYSIS AND ASSESSMENT PROCESS

GFR–Glomerular filtration rate

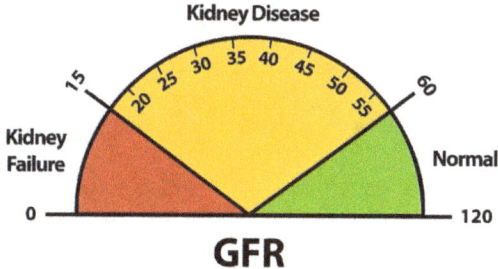

This test helps determine how much the kidney is performing. The normal range lies around 90+. The test calculates various factors, such as the patient's creatinine level, age and gender. Changes in the patient's GFR will let the doctor determine the progress.

Microalbumin

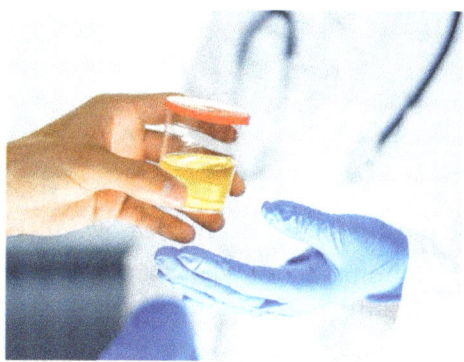

This test helps detect a protein called albumin found in the urine. It helps determine any possible kidney damage. There is no standard range as no traces of albumin must be detected.

BUN – Blood urea nitrogen

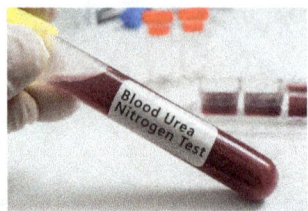

This test helps detect elevated waste levels in the blood. It serves as an early sign of reduced kidney function. The normal range is 7 to 20 milligrams per deciliter (mg/dl).

CCr – Creatinine clearance

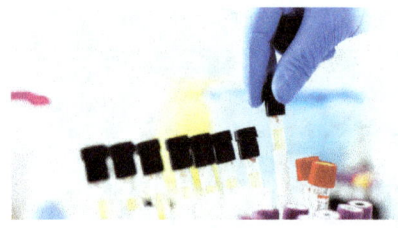

This test will help your doctor determine how much the kidneys filter creatinine and eliminate waste. For men, the normal values range from 97 to 137 milliliters per minute. In the case of women, the expected values range from 88 to 128 milliliters per minute.

Hb – Hemoglobin

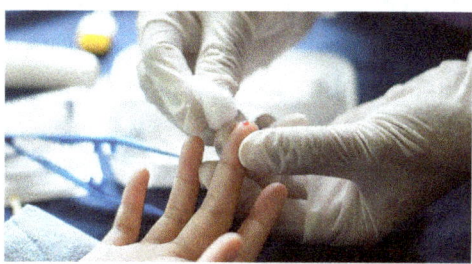

This test is important as it helps a doctor determine the hemoglobin amount in the patient's red blood cells. It also serves as a screening for anemia. In adults, the normal range lies between 12 to 18 grams per deciliter of blood.

Hct – Hematocrit

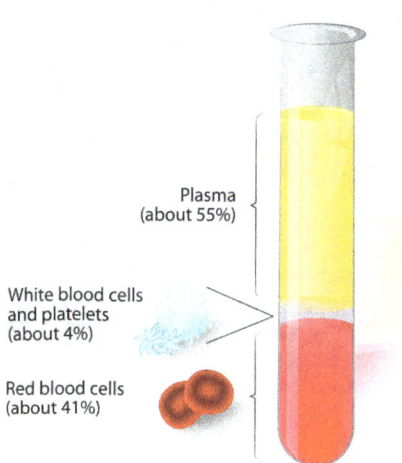

This test helps determine the percentage of red blood cells available in the bloodstream.

The normal range for women is 36% to 47%, while for males, the normal range lies between 40 to 53 percent. The hematocrit range must be kept between 33 to 36 percent in dialysis patients.

URR – Urea reduction ratio

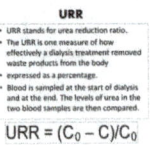

This test measures the quantity of urea removed during hemodialysis. URR should be at most 65 percent.

Kt/V

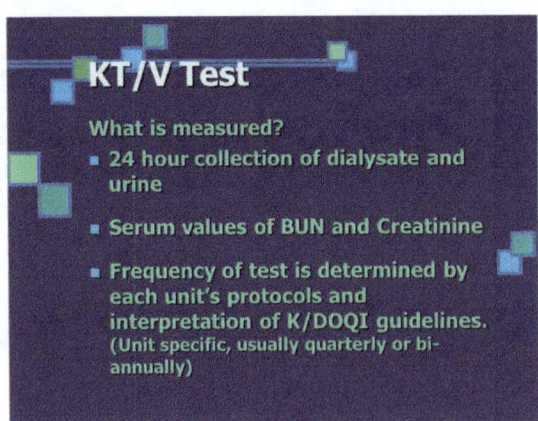

This is a mathematical formula with the following meanings:

"K" refers to clearance (the amount of urea removed by the dialyzer). This needs to be multiplied by "t" which refers to the time taken for the treatment, and this must then be divided by the "V" which refers to the volume of body fluid.

This test determines how well blood is being cleaned during dialysis. The target range must be set at more than 1.2 for hemodialysis patients, and peritoneal dialysis patients, it must be above 2.0.

A1c – Glycosylated hemoglobin test (hemoglobin A1c)

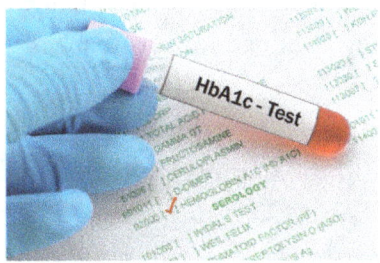

This test determines the average blood glucose levels. It is taken over a span lasting two to three months. This test is conducted for those who have diabetes.

The target range is less than 7.0 gm/dl.

Blood electrolyte levels

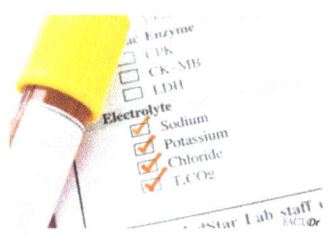

Electrolytes are essential minerals such as sodium, calcium, and potassium that prevent cardiac arrhythmia. The body gets electrolytes when consuming a healthy diet, especially whole foods. Sodium is one of the main extracellular cations in the human body and tends to affect serum osmolality significantly. Excess water in the body concerning sodium levels is standard among patients who experience severe cardiac failure. An increase in sodium levels is essential because it reduces the distance among cells, leading to significant improvements in cardiac condition, thus preventing the onset of arrhythmia. In addition, alterations in the sodium channel function have the likelihood of causing conduction disturbances that ultimately lead to cardiac arrhythmia.

Calcium is crucial in the pumping function and electrical activity that occurs in the heart. Calcium particles enter the heart's muscle cells during the heartbeat and significantly contribute to the electrical signal that conducts the coordination of the heart function. Furthermore, calcium plays an important function in regulating ionic currents and driving myofilament activation, which helps in normal electrical rhythms and prevents life-threatening arrhythmias. Normal calcium movement also prevents the impairment of the heart's relaxation or contraction, enabling normal pump function. Moreover, calcium particles are responsible for the initiation of contraction through binding to some machinery in the cells, and when this calcium binds, the cell squeezes together.

Potassium is critical in maintaining cardiovascular (CV) health and preventing arrhythmia, especially among patients at high risk of CV. Additionally, low potassium ion concentrations in the extracellular regions could alter the impacts of the antiarrhythmic drugs. The potassium ion is also the major cation found in the intracellular fluid that plays a key role in maintaining the excitability of the cell membrane. This means that a low level of serum potassium contributes to an increase in the transmembrane electrochemical gradient, consequently impairing contraction and depolarization, leading to the hyperpolarization of the cells, which is the ventricular tachyarrhythmias and no sustained ventricular tachycardias.

Magnesium is an essential electrolyte for the hydration of the cells, and the body needs it to uptake water in the cells. In addition to this, magnesium works with other minerals such as calcium, potassium, and sodium to ensure that the body has proper hydration. High levels of serum magnesium (Mg) improve the rates of survival among patients undergoing dialysis for health conditions such as end-stage renal disease (ESRD) and chronic kidney disease (CKD). Besides, high levels of serum magnesium in the body reduce the progression of CKD, while Mg supplementation reduces the progression of vascular calcification. The magnesium electrolyte can be used as a substitute for albumin among dialysis patients. This is because magnesium can provide better clinical outcomes by preventing vascular calcification from progressing.

This test measures the levels of electrolytes in the body. These are sodium, potassium, calcium and, phosphorus critical in moving nutrients and waste in and out of cells.

Here are the normal ranges:

Sodium: 135 to 145 mEq/L
Potassium: 3.5 to 5.0 mEq/L
Calcium: 8.5 to 10.5 mg/dL
Phosphorus: 3.0 to 4.5 mg/dL

Assessments a nurse needs to make the following dialysis

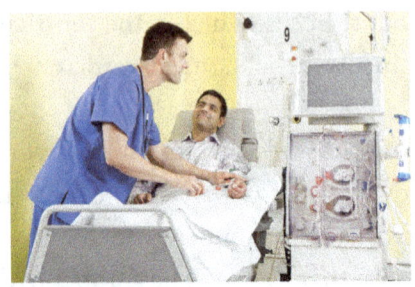

As was mentioned earlier, dialysis needs care and management even after the procedure has been performed. Once a dialysis session has been completed, the vascular access must be assessed and carefully examined for any possible signs of bleeding or hemorrhage. During moving and helping a patient being transferred to an ambulance and then to home, care must be taken to avoid trauma or exertion of pressure on the affected arm. The vascular point must also be assessed for blebs, meaning ballooning or bulging, especially any signs of an aneurysm that may lead to rupture and cause possible hemorrhage.

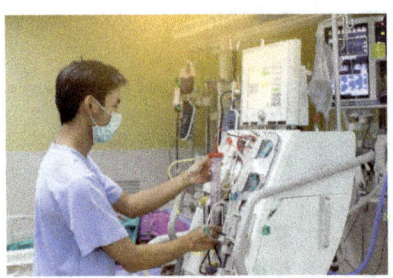

The 5 indications of hemodialysis

All nurses must be aware of these five indications when commencing dialysis. These are:

- Intractable hyperkalemia
- Acidosis
- uremic symptoms, such as nausea and malaise
- Therapy-resistant fluid overload
- CKD stage 5

Three important nursing assessments for dialysis patients

Three necessary nursing care plans that nurses must be aware of and follow for hemodialysis treatment are:

- Injury risk
- Deficient Fluid Volume
- Excess Fluid Volume

The Common complication of hemodialysis

Patients undergoing hemodialysis may suffer from acute complications during the dialysis procedure, such as intradialytic hypotension (hypertension), cardiac arrhythmias, and dialysis disequilibrium syndrome. Other complications include possible reactions to the HD membrane, bleeding, seizures, and embolism.

Role of nurses

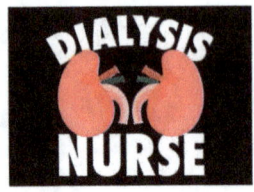

Nephrology nurses in a hemodialysis center play an important role by serving as caring individuals. Registered nurses entrusted with caring for kidney patients (nephrology nurses) have numerous responsibilities.

These are:

- To check the patients' vital signs
- Talking with patients to assess their condition
- Educating the patients about their disease
- Answering any questions asked by the patients
- Overseeing the entire dialysis treatment
- Giving patients the correct medications as advised by the doctors
- Assessing and evaluating the patients' reaction to the dialysis treatment and medications
- Reviewing of the patients' lab work
- Informing the doctors about changes in patients' conditions

CHAPTER TEN:
COMMON CAUSE OF DEATH AMONG THE DIALYSIS PATIENTS

The threat to dialysis patients increased with the emergence of the pandemic

End-stage renal disease (ESRD) is marked by a permanent decline in kidney function to the extent that renal replacement therapy becomes imperative to continue living. Though there was a decline in the mortality rate among patients afflicted with ESRD in the U.S., after 2001, the rise of Covid-19 has put ESRD patients at high risk on account of morbidity and mortality related to the pandemic. This is mainly because of the decline in immune system function and other multiple comorbidities arising from the pandemic.

The toll on the American population and economy due to ESRD

With an increase in the prevalence of ESRD, the new scenario is placing a heavy financial burden on the U.S. apart from taking a toll on the health of affected people. However, it is important to note that the current situation is far better than the dreaded scenario that existed due to ESRD 50 years ago when it was invariably lethal. Over the years, advancements in science and technology have ushered in an era of maintenance dialysis methods that have successfully served to prolong the life of ESRD patients. However, in cases of terminal uremia, the mortality rate remains high.

Though overall, an improvement in dialysis technology and a marked advance in pharmacological treatment, have been witnessed, the mortality rates among dialysis patients are relatively high and must be addressed effectively.

In the U.S., around 750,000 patients are affected by kidney failure each year, while the number across the globe is a staggering 2 million patients annually. The economic cost of sustaining life after suffering from kidney failure cannot be ignored as well. A vital stat that sheds light on the destruction of ESRD is that though the patients suffering from kidney failure only make up 1% of the total population receiving health care from the U.S. Medicaid, they still account for a whopping 7% of the total spending by Medicare.

Alternate solutions though scientifically available, still need to depict a hopeful picture. With an estimated 100,000 patients in the country on the kidney transplant list, only around 21,000 donor organs were available for transplant. The picture is all the gloomier, with the need for donor kidneys rising in the country by almost 8% annually.

ESRD affects minority and low-income groups in the U.S. more

In the U.S., Kidney failure is a condition that, apart from affecting almost 750,000 people annually, inflicts higher casualties on minority and low-income patients. Studies have shown that in comparison to the white population, African Americans, Native Americans, and Hispanics are more prone to suffer from kidney failure. The mortality rates for kidney failure treatment vary based on different factors, such as age. The mortality rate for patients after one year of treatment on dialysis is around 15 to 20% while having a 50% survival rate of five years.

Kidney failure as a global problem and comparison with the U.S.

The figures across the globe are also staggering when it comes to ESRD. According to various studies, the estimated number of people suffering from kidney failure worldwide is 2 million. At the same time, the rate at which many patients are being increasingly diagnosed with this disease continues to grow at an alarming rate of 5-7% per year among the countries with the highest prevalence of kidney failure, Taiwan, Mexico, the U.S., and Belgium top the list. Despite the lack of extensive data on worldwide mortality rates, studies dating back to 2007 showed that the mortality risk in the U.S. was 15% higher than in Europe and up to 33% higher than in Japan.

About 2.5 million people diagnosed with stage 5 chronic kidney diseases worldwide are undergoing long-term dialysis treatment. The future and prognosis of dialysis patients are not encouraging and are usually described as poor. The annual mortality rate is placed at 10% to 20%. This high mortality rate is mainly on account of cardiovascular diseases. Though statins are widely used as a pharmacological intervention, it hasn't yielded any significant results in reducing the mortality rate among dialysis patients.

Cardiovascular prevention for decreasing mortality rates among kidney failure patients

Several lifestyle recommendations have been issued for controlling the risk of mortality due to cardiovascular diseases. Among these recommendations, the most important ones are those provided by the American Heart Association for cardiovascular prevention. Among these recommendations, the most important ones are:

- Avoiding smoking
- Regular physical exercise
- Maintaining an appropriate body mass index
- Following a diet rich in fruits and vegetables
- Intake of fish
- A Diet low in salt and sugar
- Maintaining normal blood pressure
- Maintaining healthy cholesterol levels
- Maintaining glucose levels within the target

Some recommendations decrease the cardiovascular disease risk among not just the general population but also those who are on dialysis. Much of the benefits are reaped by a reduction in obesity and hypercholesterolemia. They also decrease the incidences of diabetes and hypertension. All these have been identified as key risk factors that increase the risk for cardiovascular diseases among kidney failure patients.

Survival rates for dialysis patients

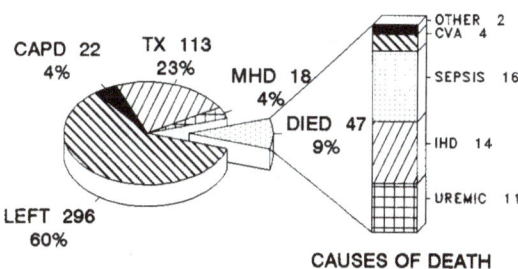

Pie-graph of the distribution percentages of co-morbid conditions that lead to mortality of ESRD

Speaking generally, the survival rates for dialysis patients are not very encouraging, with experts terming them poor. The United States Renal Data System (USRDS) reports a marked difference in the treatment of hemodialysis patients compared to those on peritoneal dialysis. The survival rate for the former stands at 57% 3 years after the patients suffered from ESKD, while the latter's, figure stands at 68% after ESKD. The survival rate after five years stands at 42% for patients receiving hemodialysis, while for those receiving peritoneal dialysis, it stands at 52%.

In this regard, it is pertinent to mention that through deceased donor kidney transplantation, the 3-year survival rate significantly climbs up to 85%. In comparison, the survival rate based on age and sex for the population stands at 92-94%. The 5-year survival of long-term dialysis patients may be either longer or shorter than cancer patients.

For the population aged 40 to 44 years, the expected life span range was approximately 8 years for dialysis patients, as the United States

Renal Data System (USRDS) report revealed. For the age group between 60-64 years, the expected life span range was approximately 4.5 years.

Factors that are closely associated with survival chances of the dialysis patients

A few factors closely associated with dialysis patients survival chances are discussed below.

Patient Demographics

Studies and research have established that the survival rates for patients start to decline with increasing age. Also, it has been found with evidence that among the age group who are less than 45 years old, males tend to do better as compared to females. However, the outlook changes after individuals turn above 65 as then the males are found to have a lower adjusted mortality rate.

As far as mortality rates among the other age groups are concerned, the rates are not constant. However, research has shown that Asian Americans and African-Americans tend to have better survival rates when comparing these groups with the Caucasian groups.

Dialysis Vintage

Dialysis vintage means the length of time on dialysis, and it is an important factor in the mortality of patients suffering from ESKD. The time since initiation of dialysis is an important factor that cannot be ignored. The mortality rate drops initially for those who have been put on hemodialysis, reaching its lowest point during Year 2. After the second year, it witnesses a continuous rise. However, this dip is not witnessed among the patients who have been put on peritoneal dialysis. Instead, evidence has shown that the rate tends to increase after initiation.

Even though research and statistics suggest a decrease in mortality among kidney failure patients on hemodialysis by the year 2, the initial 3 months are classified as a period of high risk starting on hemodialysis.

Dialysis Modality – comparing hemodialysis with peritoneal dialysis

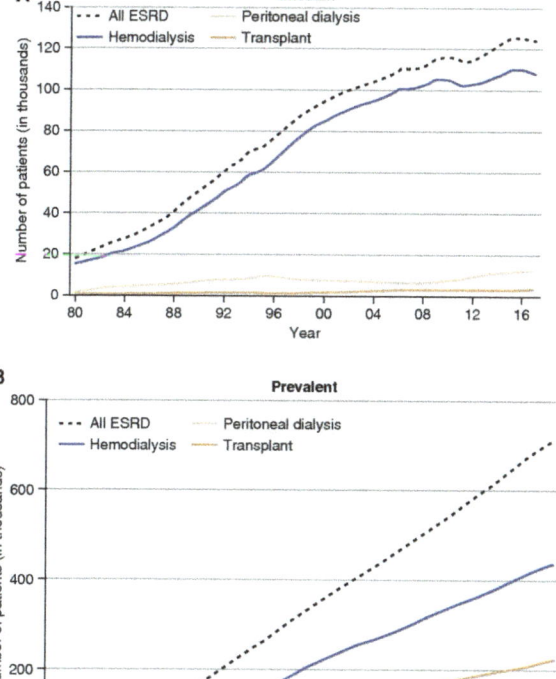

Detailed data regarding these two modalities still needs to be included, but still, there is previous observational data available. This available data supports peritoneal dialysis regarding the mortality rate in the first years of treatment. However, after the second year, the advantage shifts comparatively to hemodialysis. To explain this change in observation, it can be concluded that there is a better preservation of residual kidney function in the initial years of treatment of patients undergoing peritoneal dialysis. However, the ultrafiltration capacity then falls in the coming years, which is why in terms of mortality, peritoneal dialysis has yet to have an advantage after two years.

In contrast, since there are other factors, such as sicker patients and the need to start hemodialysis urgently, the early treatment period tends to have a much higher initial mortality rate. It is also necessary to note that sicker patients are treated almost exclusively with HD.

The most common cause of high mortality among ESRD patients undergoing dialysis

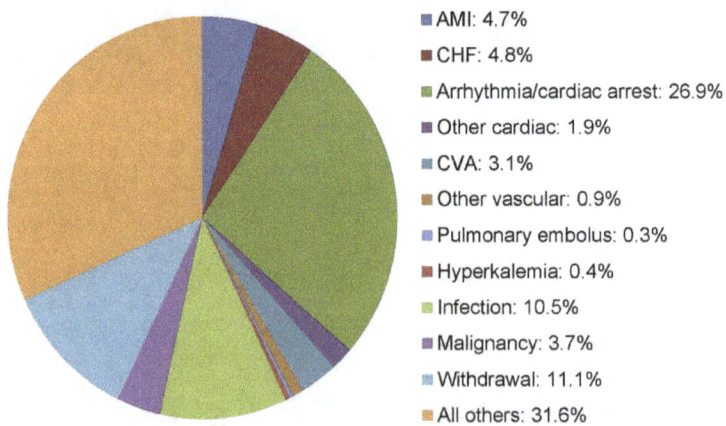

Figure: Arrhythmia and Sudden Death in Hemodialysis Patients: Protocol and Baseline Characteristics of the Monitoring in Dialysis Study

As discussed above, patients suffering from ESKD are at an increased risk due to the burden of cardiovascular disease, which significantly impacts their life and outlook. The risk of cardiovascular disease factor is much higher when comparing these patients to the general population. Among the various cardiac conditions found in ESKD patients, the most common one is coronary artery disease. Statistics suggest that CVD is the leading cause of death among dialysis patients.

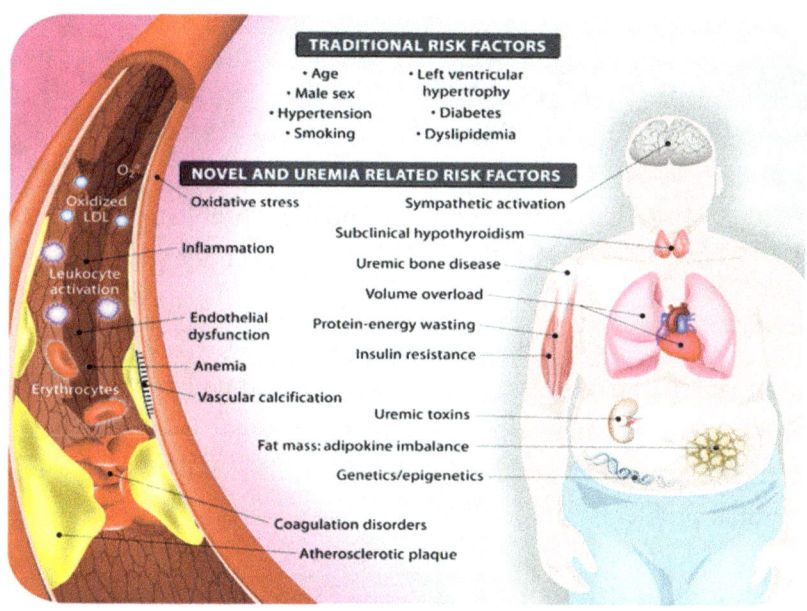

Figure: Emerging Biomarkers for Evaluating Cardiovascular Risk in the Chronic Kidney Disease Patient: How Do New Pieces Fit into the Uremic Puzzle?

When summarizing the overall mortality rate, the burden of cardiovascular disease is the most critical factor behind the cause of death and its effect on life expectancy in the maintenance of dialysis patients. The mortality rate is 10-20 times higher among dialysis patients than in the general population. The risk stands at the highest in the initial 120 days after dialysis has been initiated. The annual mortality is around 9% annually with 40-50% 5-year survival. As mentioned above, cardiovascular disease is the leading cause of the death of dialysis patients. Hence, following the recommendations mentioned above in this chapter is crucial to increase life longevity. The next major cause of death is on account of an infectious complication. Other than that, the studies available have suggested comparable outcomes for the two different types of dialysis.

Uremic pruritus and associated factors in hemodialysis patients

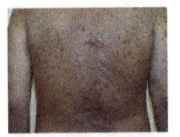

Uremic pruritus is a medical problem that is very common among ESRD patients undergoing dialysis. Closely linked with health-related quality impairments, it is experienced by almost half dialysis patients. It has also been independently associated with mortality. This problem is still being studied, and its pathogenesis has yet to be entirely understood by experts. However, it is known that it is a multifactorial problem.

Statistics show that ESRD patients are commonly afflicted by severe pruritus. Though its pathogenesis remains unknown, it has been established that improving dialysis quality helps reduce the prevalence and severity of this problem. Other methods beneficial for this condition include topical and systemic agents. Broadband ultraviolet phototherapy is also helpful. Another effective agent that alleviates the severity is gabapentin among ESRD pruritus patients. Among other options being explored are Kappa opiate agonists that show promising results.

Causes of uremic pruritus

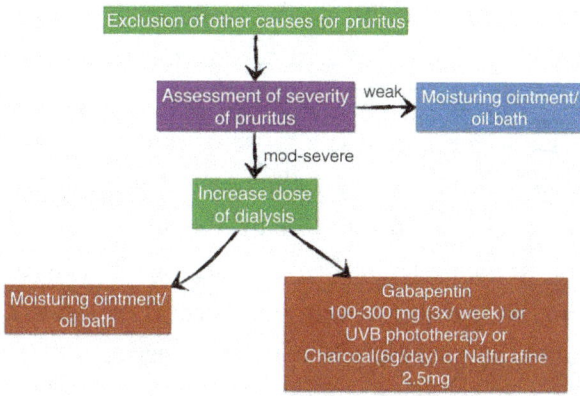

Figure: **Uremic Pruritis - Algorithm for Management**

Certain triggering factors, such as uremia-related abnormalities are believed to be the root cause. These abnormalities involve calcium, phosphorus, and parathyroid hormone metabolism. Other causes that trigger this condition are an accumulation of uraemic toxins or systemic inflammation. Cutaneous xerosis may also trigger this condition, while common co-morbidities, including diabetes mellitus and viral hepatitis, are also recognized as the causes.

Pruritus and link with death

Uremic pruritus produces unwanted effects and is an unpleasant complication in dialysis patients. Patients undergoing maintenance dialysis (MHD) suffer from this condition commonly. As mentioned above, though the pathogenesis and etiology of this condition are not known as of now, experts cite this as a multifactorial condition. The prevalence of this condition is high, standing at 22% to 90%. It has been found to impact the patient's quality of life negatively and is linked to death.

As discussed in the above section in this chapter, cardiovascular disease and infection-related deaths are the leading causes of high mortality rates in dialysis patients. Research has shown that uremic pruritus is a presentation of systemic inflammation. Experts have concluded that this systemic inflammation is a cause of cardiovascular mortality in hemodialysis patients. However, there are other causes too that lead to cardiovascular disease. It is important to note that, at present, studies that explore the correlation between pruritus and mortality of HD patients are not available in large numbers. There is also a lack of sufficient studies that explore the correlation between cardiovascular or infection-related mortality and this condition.

Nephrologists and related healthcare workers need to adopt caution and address the cardiovascular risks in hemodialysis patients in case the patient is also suffering from Uremic pruritus. Deaths on account of infection have also been found to be more prevalent in patients suffering from severe uremic pruritus when such patients are compared with other groups.

The future course of action

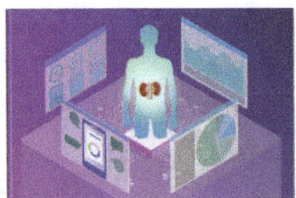

ESRD is a major cause of concern to society and the country, on the whole, owing to its high morbidity and mortality rates. It also has significant social and financial implications, which makes it a major public health problem that needs to be addressed. The outcome of this disease depends mainly on several factors, such as different treatment modalities (hemodialysis and peritoneal dialysis). However, other important factors also need to be considered, like co-morbidities, age, and duration of dialysis. Other factors that have an outcome are the role of supportive therapies and the successful implementation of infection control strategies.

CHAPTER ELEVEN:
DIALYZABLE MEDICATIONS

Medication to avoid or adjust before and during dialysis

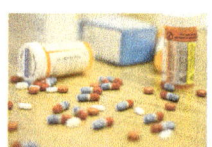
Similar to other forms of medical treatment procedures, medications need to be avoided or adjusted before continuing with the dialysis process. Among the many things to consider, medications are an important aspect that cannot be ignored. This is because administering some drugs before commencing dialysis may cause severe health risks of the patient's health. Hence, it becomes essential to check the medications that are being given before and during the treatment.

For patients put on dialysis, here are the following medications that need to be avoided during the dialysis treatment:

- Blood pressure medications
- Antibiotic medications

Apart from these two classes of medications, other medications may need to be avoided depending on different factors.

Why is there a need to hold medications for dialysis

The issue with medications is that the dialysis process works by filtering and cleansing the blood, similar to how a kidney works. Hence, the process of dialysis may result in the medications being dialyzed. This means that the medications that are taken before the dialysis procedure may become ineffective. Hence, such medications need to be avoided.

Since patients with kidney failure require dialysis treatment, it is essential to sometimes hold the blood pressure medicines. This is because taking BP medications will drop the blood pressure further, and the patient may have a low BP during dialysis. To avoid this scenario, patients on dialysis may be required to quit their blood pressure medications during dialysis frequently.

Anticoagulant drugs given to patients during dialysis

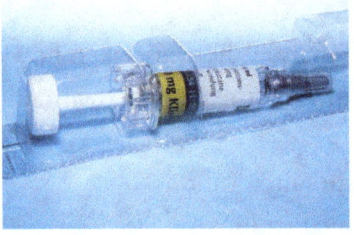

Two main anticoagulant drugs given to patients during hemodialysis treatment are heparin and enoxaparin. These are required to prevent the blood from clotting. Preventing blood clotting when it is filtered through the dialysis machine (artificial kidney) is important and a part of kidney failure management.

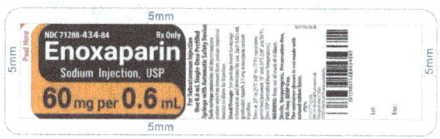

These anticoagulant drugs help prevent coagulation, also known as blood clotting, by inhibiting Vitamin K production in the liver. These drugs increase the time it takes for the blood to clot. Although some healthcare professionals refer to these drugs as blood thinners, it is important to note that they do not thin the blood. These drugs cannot dissolve clots that have already formed. However, these drugs will prevent an existing clot from enlarging further.

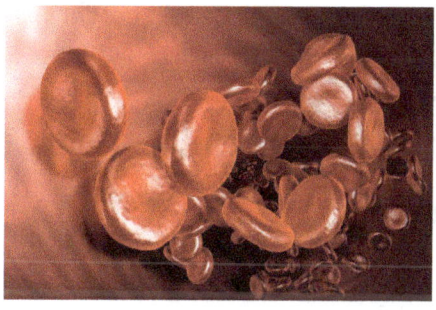

It is essential to note the complications while taking these drugs with other medicines. This is because some medicines interfere with anticoagulants. The medicines that are used for preventing and treating blood clots may interfere with these drugs. The same is the case with medicines that contain aspirin or salicylates. Another medicine known as Dextran 40, used to treat shock, also interferes with these drugs. Hence, it becomes important to avoid these complications. Also, medicines used for treating inflammatory disease may interfere with anticoagulant drugs. Examples are oral corticosteroids and non-steroidal anti-inflammatory medicines.

A dialysis patient using these anticoagulants may need to exercise some precautions. It is best to ask the doctor about any activities, such as sports, that may need to be stopped. Exercising precaution is necessary because, at times, there may be internal bleeding due to an injury without the individual even realizing it.

It is also important to inform your doctor if an individual experiences the following symptoms:

- Difficulty breathing
- Fainting
- Itchy hives
- Hay fever
- Blisters
- Symptoms of allergy
- Bleeding from the nose
- Prolonged bleeding due to cuts
- Urine that is red or brown
- Numbness
- Difficulty in coordination
- Blurred vision
- Dizziness
- Confusion
- Severe abdominal pain
- Headache
- Rask on mouth or eyes
- Chest pain
- White or blue color evident in toes or fingers

Dialyzable medicines and the mechanism of being dialyzed in the dialysis machine

What does it exactly mean when it is said that medication is dialyzable? It means that the medicine is capable of being dialyzed. In terms of dialysis, it means that the medicine can diffuse through a dialyzing membrane.

How to find out if a drug is dialyzable?

To determine whether a drug is dialyzable, few basic rules aid in determining whether the drug is dialyzable. In this regard, the size of the molecules in medicine matters a lot. The dialysis machine efficiently cleared molecules with low molecular weight, like less than 500 Daltons. Larger molecules or weight compounds that have a high molecular weight, like greater than 2000 Daltons, are not cleared.

Meaning of not dialyzable

A not dialyzable drug means it cannot be removed undergoing to dialysis.

Properties that make a drug more dialyzable

Some drugs are easily cleared, while others are not. As a general rule, drugs with a small molecular size and small volume of distribution are easily cleared by dialysis. High water solubility is another property that makes it easy to clear drugs through dialysis.

Dialysis and physicochemical characteristics of the drug

What Determines Drug Dialyzability?
- molecular size,
- Protein binding,
- volume of distribution,
- water solubility,
- plasma clearance
- Dialysis Membrane (Pore size, surface Area)
- Blood and Dialysate Flow Rates

The extent to which a drug taken would be affected by dialysis depends on its different physicochemical characteristics. Here is a brief discussion of these characteristics.

Molecular size

Molecular size is important in determining how the dialysis procedure would affect the drug. Drugs with smaller molecular weight substances can be dialyzed easily; these molecules pass easily through the dialysis membrane, while drugs with greater molecular size would not.

Protein binding

Protein binding plays an integral part in dialysis as drug-protein complexes that are too large would be unable to cross the dialysis membrane.

Volume of distribution

This implies that drugs with an extensive distribution volume would be subjected to minimal dialysis.

Water solubility

Some drugs have high water solubility while some have low. Hence, the drugs possessing high water solubility will be easily dialyzed to a greater extent. In contrast, drugs that do not have high water solubility or ones with high lipid solubility will be dialyzed to a lesser extent.

Dialysis Membrane

Another characteristic that has an important effect on the dialysis of a drug is the dialysis procedure's technical aspects. Earlier in this chapter, the dialysis membrane was mentioned and how small molecules can pass through it. However, there is a lot more to it. The dialysis of a drug does not merely depend on the different physicochemical characteristics of a drug. It also depends on the dialysis membrane's characteristics. These refer to the dialysis membrane's pore size, surface area, and geometry. All these aspects play a crucial role in defining the extent of the dialysis of drugs.

Dialysis flow rates

The dialysis flow rates are also an important factor affecting drug dialysis. If the drug concentration is low, dialysis can be significantly achieved, even if the dialysate flow rate is faster. However, if the drug concentration is decreased, the flow rate would need to be lowered to achieve a greater level of dialysis.

An important fact that is worthy of mention here is that the peritoneal membrane used in peritoneal dialysis is larger than the dialysis membrane used in hemodialysis.

List of common dialyzable medicines

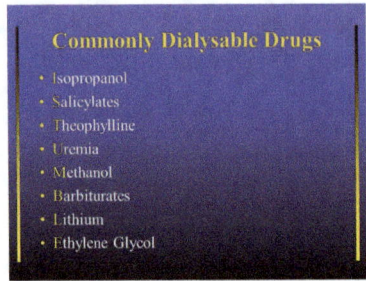

- Barbiturates
- Lithium
- Isoniazid
- Salicylates
- Theophylline/Caffeine (methylxanthines)
- Methanol
- Metformin
- Ethylene glycol
- Depakote
- Dabigatran
- Carbamazepine
- INH/isopropyl alcohol
- Salicylates
- Theophylline
- Uremia
- Methanol
- Barbiturates
- Lithium

- Ethylene glycol
- Dabigatran
- Depakote

Reasons why antibiotics are given after dialysis

Giving antibiotics after dialysis becomes important for different reasons, especially for patients suffering from end-stage renal disease. Administering IV antibiotics to patients following intermittent hemodialysis is necessary because antibiotics improve the patient's convenience.

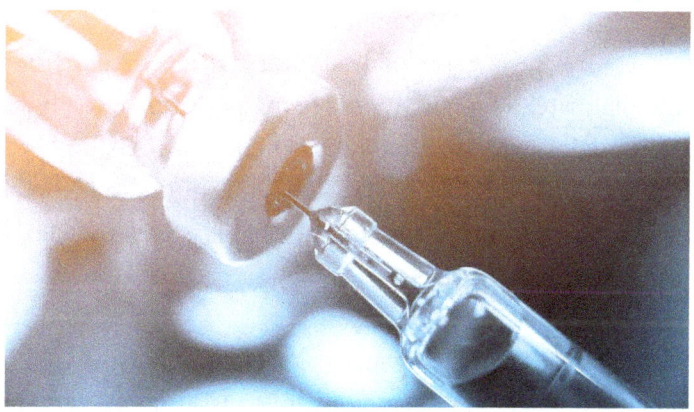

Antibiotics also reduce the risk of contracting infections and help avoid thrombotic complications. The infection risk among dialysis patients is very high because such patients have an impaired immune system. Also, such patients require frequent use of catheters or may need needles inserted in their veins to access their bloodstream for dialysis. In such cases, it becomes vital to minimize the risk of infection by giving antibiotics.

These antibiotics also help reduce the healthcare costs that would otherwise be incurred due to the placement of an additional CVC (central venous access).

The different types of dialyzers

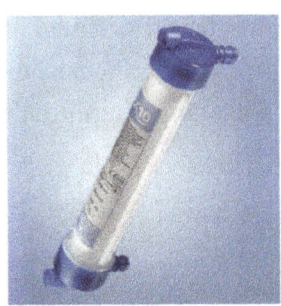

Different dialyzers, known as Artificial Kidneys, are required by patients suffering from kidney failure to clean their blood and remove fluids. The dialyzer comprises a dialysis membrane supported by a structure that functions as a kidney and act as a replacement. Dialysis is an essential part of the dialyzer. It is used to separate the blood from the dialysate. When dialysis is being performed, the blood and dialysate flow in opposite directions. The flow occurs on both sides of the membrane. This allows for water and solutes to be exchanged through the semi-permeable membrane. This is how the need for an artificial kidney is fulfilled.

The dialyzer's performance gauges the effectiveness of the dialysis treatment.. The dialyzer's characteristics consist of two parts, known as the design characteristics and the functional characteristics. The dialyzer's design features are:

- The configuration of the dialyzer
- The pre-charge of the blood chamber
- Dialysate chamber
- The type of membrane
- The biocompatibility

On the other hand, the working characteristics refer to the transfer rate of water and different solutes. Different classification methods for dialyzers exist in different parts of the world. They are mentioned below:

Classification of dialyzers based on dialyzer's configuration

Three types come to the fore when dialyzers are classified based on their configuration. They are:

- Tube type
- Flat type
- and hollow fiber type

Currently, all over the globe, the most commonly used dialyzer is the hollow fiber type, while the other two types of dialyzers that were used in the past are no longer utilized for dialysis.

The hollow fiber dialyzer, which is in use currently, consists of around 8000-12000 hollow fibers. The fiber has an inner diameter of about 200-300um with a wall thickness of around 2-30um. This type of dialyzer has its hollow fibers bundled into bundles. These bundles are placed to form a dialyzer casing. The casing, along with the dialyzing membrane, is both sealed by using polyurethane. The blood is made to flow through the hollow fibers, while the dialysate is made to flow in the opposite direction outside the fibers.

Classification of dialyzers based on the dialyzer's membrane material

Based on this classification method, the dialyzers are divided into four different parts. They are discussed below:

Regenerated cellulose membrane dialyzer

This type of dialyzer includes two important components, known as the copper imitation membrane and the copper ammonia membrane dialyzer, with free hydroxyl groups preened on the surface of the cellulose membrane. These react with the blood components and are generally deemed to poor biocompatibility. However, after treatment, the fiber surface becomes smoother while the biocompatibility is enhanced.

Acetate cellulose membrane dialyzer

To improve the biocompatibility of this dialyzer and its performance, the cellulose membrane is acetylated so that the film is formed.

Replacing the fiber membrane dialyzer

Using the blood imitation membrane serves as an alternative copper imitation membrane. It has surface-free hydroxyl groups that are covered by tertiary ammonia compounds. These compounds offer good biocompatibility.

Synthetic fiber membrane dialyzer

Different materials are used in this type of dialyzer. These are polyacrylonitrile, polymethylmethacrylate, and polysulfone. Other materials used include polycarbonate, polyethylene, and polyamide.

These materials offer a high transport and ultrafiltration coefficient that improves biocompatibility. However, this type of dialyzer comes with an expensive cost.

Classification of dialyzers based on the dialyzer's ultrafiltration coefficient

According to this type of classification, dialyzers can be divided into two types. These are discussed below:

Low ultrafiltration coefficient dialyzer

This type of dialyzer has an ultrafiltration coefficient of <15ml/mmHg. It consists of a copper imitation membrane, a cuprammonium membrane, and a blood imitation membrane. It also has a cellulose acetate membrane.

High-throughput and high-efficiency dialyzer

This type of dialyzer has an ultrafiltration coefficient> 15 ml/(mmHg.hm^2). It offers a very high removal rate for substances with medium molecular weight. It can remove the large molecular weight of β2-microgulobulin and other macromolecular substances.

CHAPTER TWELVE:
DIALYSIS PATIENTS BATTLING WITH MENTAL HEALTH ISSUES

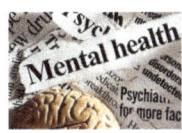

Stress is a normal faced by kidney patients

Stress is a part of human life, but the problem is that high-stress levels can impact overall health, primarily, by increasing blood pressure and causing kidney damage. Nevertheless, what if an individual's kidneys are already damaged? What if the individual is on dialysis? In such a case, managing stress and adopting coping strategies to keep it under control to prevent further kidney damage becomes important.

Stress in brief

Stress is defined as any factor that has the potential to upset or disturb an individual's mental and emotional balance. It can be induced by physiological factors, such as injury, infection, or disease, or by psychological means, such as anxiety, conflict, and threats. On the other hand, patients facing kidney failure or kidney disease can find this problem contributing to stress. The very breaking of news that an individual has a chronic illness, like kidney disease, can elevate stress levels.

Psychological stress is inevitable for most people as they have to contend with it almost every other day. Such stress may be induced in both positive and negative ways. Positive life events, like marriage and children, may bring about this effect, and even emotionally challenging events that are hard to digest, like the loss of a loved one or financial problems, cause stress.

Stress is typical in most cases, and the body's response to such a threat usually manifests as an increase in heart rate, faster breathing, elevated blood pressure, and tense muscles. These responses are natural and a part of the body's mechanisms. Stress also causes an increase in blood sugar and blood fat levels. Almost every individual has studied the body's response to stress in terms of "fight or flight." It would be safe to suggest that such responses are a part of the natural process that helps the individual face and survive immediate dangers. However, these reactions result in high or constant stress in the long run. This will eventually take its toll on the individual's health.

Impact of stress on kidneys

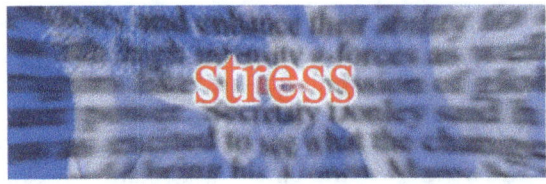

While the body's reaction to stress is benefits individuals as it prepares them to confront immediate dangers or looming crises, it also serves as a positive motivator. This implies that it helps an individual handle life's challenges if the energy is used positively and appropriately channeled. However, the situation will slowly change if the human body is made to endure high-stress levels continuously. In such a case, these physical reactions, if allowed to persist continuously, will eventually cause harm to the health. These will be felt in several ways, such as increased blood pressure and a faster heart rate combined with higher fat and sugar levels in the blood. All these will contribute to increasing the health problems in the body, such as hypertension, diabetes, and cardiovascular disease.

Stress for extended periods can also cause damage to the kidneys. Kidneys are prone to problems with the blood circulatory system; hence, the blood vessels, and the filtering units, need to function properly. People who encounter high levels of stress are at an increased risk of suffering from high blood pressure and diabetes are hence susceptible to kidney disease. While kidney disease also causes the patient to be at high risk for heart and blood vessel disease. If the individual suffers from heart and blood vessel disease combined with kidney disease, stress can ignite a dangerous reaction in the body. Hence, managing stress and keeping it under control becomes extremely important if an individual wants to prevent heart and kidney disease. It also becomes necessary if the individual wants to maintain their overall health if they are already diagnosed with heart and kidney disease.

Managing stress

Avoiding and eliminating stress in full may not be possible so physical reaction to stress will always be present. However, the important thing to consider is that some steps can be taken to manage and keep stress control, especially the body's response to stress. Here are a few tips to control stress if you already have an ailing condition, such as heart disease or kidney disease:

- Intake of healthy foods
- Limiting the intake of salt
- Limiting the use of caffeine
- Limiting sugar intake
- Spending time relaxing
- Practicing relaxation techniques
- Talking to a loved one, healthcare professional, or friend
- Writing down your problems on a piece of paper and figuring out the solution
- Setting realistic goals and modest expectations
- Sleeping for 7 to 8 hours
- Being optimistic
- Going on a vacation
- Exercising regularly

Uremic Toxins Build up after discontinuing Dialysis

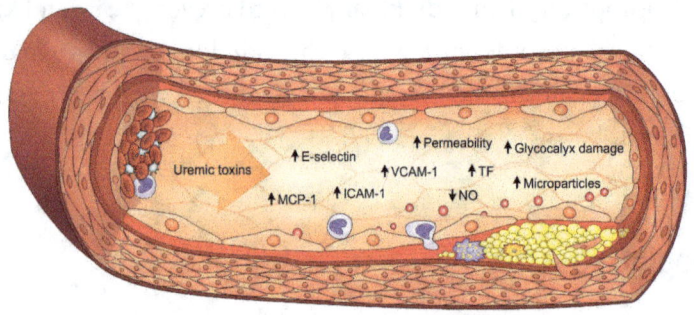

Stopping dialysis leads to toxins building up in the bloodstream. This eventually leads to a condition known as uremia. The patient will then require medicines for managing uremia symptoms and other underlying medical conditions. Death occurs within a few days or after a few weeks after the toxins start building up in the body. The speed of death depends on how fast the toxins build up in the body.

Effects of Uremic Toxins on human body

The buildup of toxins causes a person to face specific physical and emotional changes. As a few days pass, the human body is on its way to shut down. Prior to this shutdown, a series of changes occurred in the body that are mentioned below:

- Loss of appetite
- Loss of fluid overload
- Sleeping a lot
- Restlessness
- Disorientation
- Confusion
- Failure to recognize people previously known
- Changes in breathing
- Congestion
- Changes in color

Medicines are available for symptoms, like pain, anxiety, or congestion. After the body's systems shut down, the person falls unconscious, and the heart eventually stops functioning.

Altered mental status caused due to high blood glucose levels

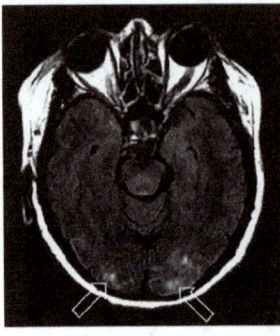

Altered mental status (AMS) is a disruption caused by brain functioning that leads to behavioral change. The change may occur suddenly and take some time. This problem varies from individual to individual, ranging from slight confusion in a mental state to total disorientation. It may also lead to sleepiness and coma.

The onset of AMS is marked by any of the following physical, psychological, and environmental factors:

- Low sugar levels
- High blood sugar levels
- Diabetic ketoacidosis
- History of high blood pressure, diabetes
- Psychiatric illness

Signs and symptoms

Here are some of the most common signs:

- Lack of concentration
- Forgetfulness
- Slow response to a situation
- Hallucinations
- Changes in sleep patterns
- Decreased or increased movement
- Agitation

- Rambling speech
- Difficulty waking up from sleep

AMS treatment

Treatment usually depends on the cause. Treatments may be required using oxygen and medicines. These will help alleviate the symptoms. In case of severe symptoms, hospitalization may be required.

Treatment options

The following medications are a part of the treatment process:

Hydergine, Haldol, haloperidol, Fanapt, and Haldol Decanoate.

High glucose levels and infection

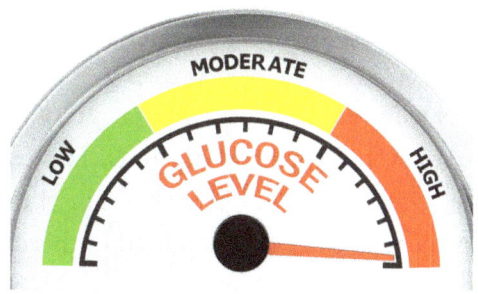

Elevated blood sugar levels cause harm to the body. It primarily impairs the body's natural immune defenses. It also increases the risk of contracting many viral, fungal, bacterial, and parasitic infections. The condition marked by increased blood glucose following a new infection aggravates the symptoms.

Experts recommend controlling glucose levels as they impact the immune system defenses. Diabetes over a prolonged period may result in peripheral nerve damage. It reduces blood flow to the extremities, increasing infection chances.

Frequent high blood sugar levels over time cause permanent damage to body parts. These include the kidneys, eyes, nerves, and blood vessels.

Impact of aging Factors like Dementia, Depression, Cognitive Decline on mental health of dialysis patients

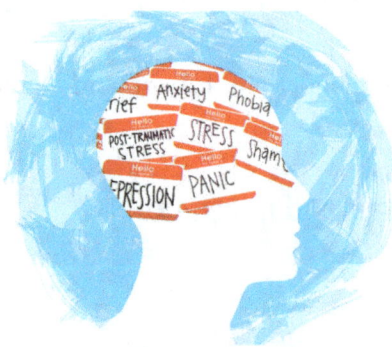

Experts regard chronic kidney disease as a multifaceted condition with physical and psychological implications. This is why managing such an issue requires a multidisciplinary team effort. The help of mental health professionals may be required in this case, who would collaborate with nephrologists to implement measures necessary for the holistic management of this condition. Those who suffer from kidney disease or renal failure and require dialysis exhibit signs of psychological problems. The treatment methods of such individuals will vary from person to person and need to conform individually. At times, medications may be required to manage such patients.

Since dialysis patients have an all-out dependence on a machine for life, it will take a toll on their health. No other medical condition requires such an abject dependence on continuous treatment to stay alive. The maintenance treatment of a chronic illness like kidney failure has severe repercussions on the mental health of such patients. Dialysis turns out to be a procedure that is extremely stressful for the patient. The situation aggravates if there is a lack of proper education and preparation to deal with a condition like ESRD.

Depression

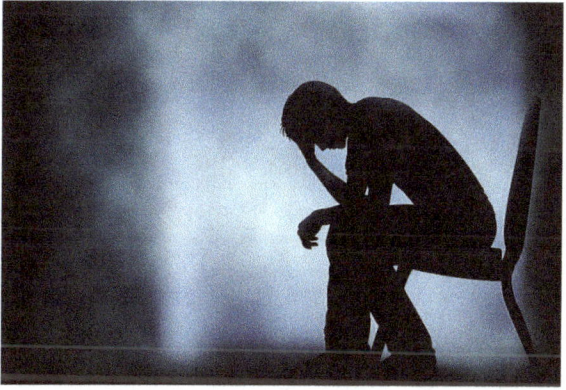

This condition is one of the most common psychiatric complications that arises in a patient suffering from renal failure. One condition that aggravates the situation is that most dialysis patients fail to return to work and earn indepedently. Work is not only necessary as a source of income, but it induces positive emotions, such as a sense of accomplishment, and boosts self-esteem. Missing out on a job makes a patient vulnerable to depression. Depression may need to be treated with medications, such as an antidepressant therapy and psychotherapy.

Suicidal behavior

When a patient suffers from extreme depression, the threat of suicide always looms large. Hence, the issue of suicidal behavior comes among dialysis patients. Many observational studies have linked dialysis to high suicide rates as compared to the average healthy population. The problem is all the more serious because missing dialysis can result in death.

Delirium

Electrolyte imbalance is a common condition following dialysis and is called dialysis disequilibrium syndrome. It may also result due to medical or surgical complications. This condition, such has different reasons, such as anemia, uremia, and hyperparathyroidism.

Also, there is the threat of dementia present among the elderly with diabetes and receiving dialysis. Dementia has different reasons, such as Alzheimer's disease and dialysis dementia syndrome. It may also have vascular causes.

Mood swings

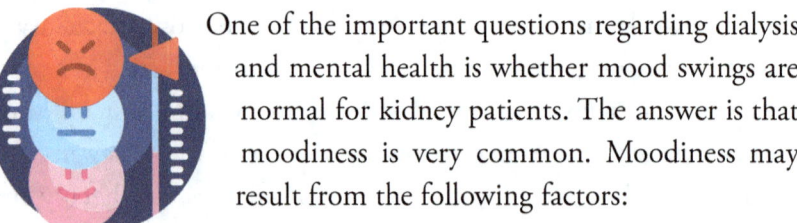

One of the important questions regarding dialysis and mental health is whether mood swings are normal for kidney patients. The answer is that moodiness is very common. Moodiness may result from the following factors:

- Uremia, or the waste products accumulating in the bloodstream, irritates the nervous system, leading to increased

irritability. This usually happens in the initial days after being diagnosed with kidney disease
- Medications also cause moodiness while making some people depressed

The problem is that the stress endured due to a chronic illness affects the mood and feelings, causing different symptoms, such as irritability, anger, and frustration due to the overwhelming nature of the illness. Feelings of hopelessness and helplessness are also common when faced with a life-threatening disease that requires being dependent on a machine for a lifetime.

The role of Dialysis Team Members and need for Family Support to help dialysis patients

Ask any renal patient and those on dialysis, and you will discover that such patients have to endure numerous stresses and frustrations due to this medical condition. This situation may be very difficult at times. Even the patient's loved ones and close ones of the patient may feel the toll. The case becomes more complicated if the patient and family members have yet to witness such a situation before. An unexpected prognosis will also further aggravate the situation and increase the suffering.

In such times, helplessness is prevalent because they cannot do anything about it. There may be a fear of the consequences of this medical condition. A mark of such a situation or gravity starts affecting everyone. As everyone, from the patient to the family members, try to cope with the situation and fulfill the demands of dialysis, it may lead to a rise in anxiety while everyday life may be disrupted. What usually follows is scrutinizing the dialysis team members and the health care system. Hence, the role of the dialysis team members becomes essential.

> **Dialysis Health Care Team**
> - Patient
> - Dialysis Nurse
> - Dialysis Technician
> - Nephrologist
> - Nephrology Social Worker
> - Renal Dietitian

Kidney failure is a condition that necessitates lifestyle changes. A huge change marks it as routine activities that earlier required minor physical exertion now become an arduous tasks. Family members and close friends must be responsible role by taking on some responsibilities to help the patient. The good news is that with proper treatment, family life may return to normal to a great extent.

Here are a few steps that the family members and the dialysis team members can take to lessen the stress:

- Discussing the issues with the dialysis staff, including doctors
- Write down issues being faced and seek solutions
- The Dialysis unit must inform family members about any changes required in patient's treatment

- Educate yourself more about the illness through credible resources
- Engage in pleasures and activities that lift the mood
- Staying responsible for daily activities
- Exercising to maintain physical health
- Sharing feelings with family and trusted friends
- Discussing feelings with other patients
- Seeking extra help from other sources too, such as a social worker involved in dialysis work or an outside counselor
- Make sure all family or personal problems are addressed
- Keeping your previous goals in mind, try arranging treatment in ways that will allow the individual to accomplish all goals
- Exercise patience
- Setting realistic goals while adjusting to the required lifestyle changes

Opting for professional counseling

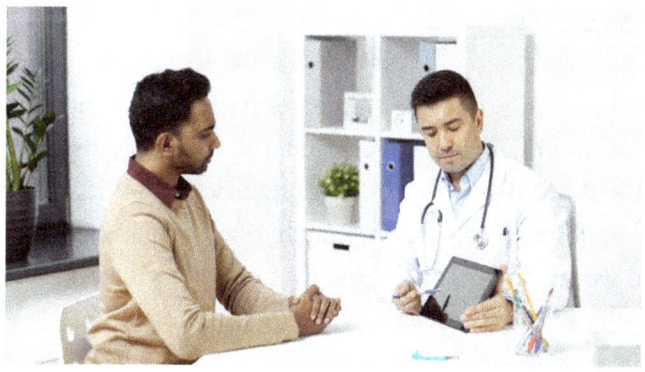

Living with kidney disease and undergoing its treatment can be very upsetting, especially in the initial weeks and months. The news of kidney disease and the need to be on dialysis can make the patients and their families delve into grieving as they make changes to adjust to the new requirements. This could be when patients and their family members undergo complex feelings. The family and dialysis team members have an important responsibility to help the patient navigate through such changes.

This is the time when the patient needs to seek for professional counseling services. Usually, dialysis units are equipped with trained counselors and clinical social workers who can offer adjustment counseling. A patient needs counseling if they present the following symptoms:

- Depression that lasts more than two weeks
- Thoughts about committing suicide
- Loss or increase in appetite
- Sleeping little or more
- Losing interest in activities that the patient usually enjoyed
- Angry outbursts
- Drug, alcohol, or substance abuse
- Inability to make major decisions
- Social withdrawal

Counseling helps greatly as it prepares patients and their families to learn ways to utilize their inner strengths and apply them to benefit from new ways of coping with kidney disease and its treatment. A local mental health professional, such as a psychiatrist, psychologist, or social worker, can help. Asking for help through counseling is not and should not be considered a sign of weakness.

Impact of dialysis on mental health of patients and the role of nurse

Renal nurses in a dialysis setting may encounter challenging and stressful situations because patients receiving dialysis treatment are forced to live with high levels of severe stress that force them to adopt and display behaviors that may be termed hostile. However, managing such behavior while completing the treatment is important and necessary for the patient' safety and the institute's image. Generally speaking, nurses in a dialysis setting and those dealing with kidney patients are trained regarding the technical aspects of dialysis and have limited knowledge and training to provide only a minimal level of psychological support, since they are not trained to manage patients exhibiting signs of severe mental stress, it becomes important to be a good self-learner and enhance professional development by being a quick and sharp observer.

There are generally four main areas of interest for nurses where they need to play an active role. In terms of patient's benefits, these areas are:

- Patient and staff safety concerns
- Facilitating care
- Educating
- Supporting the needs of patients

It does not come as a surprise that renal nurses and those involved in assisting in the dialysis treatment may find difficulty and face tough challenges in managing the hostile and disturbed behavior demonstrated by patients on dialysis who have significant levels of stress or display signs of severe mental illness. However, in most settings, despite the unprecedented difficulties facing nurses, most of these professionals adopt a person-centered approach that helps them navigate through such tough situations through informed measures directed at to ensure patient safety.

However, nurses also encounter other challenges in the treatment setting. These include but are not limited to staff shortages and lack of training. These problems hinder specialized care delivery and may affect treatment outcomes, making the situation more stressful for the patients and their families. To encounter such problems, attention must be paid to addressing such issues, and the related resources must be allocated to avoid such a situation from impacting treatment outcomes or even hurting the image of the healthcare institute. Education on mental health illnesses is necessary for nurses. Nurses should take the initiative to arm themselves with this knowledge critical to assisting patients on dialysis. This way, the treatment outcomes can be improved significantly, benefiting patient, their families, and the healthcare staff.

In addition, support from senior staff and increased collaboration with other healthcare workers of the dialysis team can help nurses be better prepared for patient treatment. It will help instill in them a feeling of confidence. It will also enhance and boost nurses' knowledge and experience in dealing with such issues. All such measures will help the patients navigate these difficult times with easily and comfortably.

CHAPTER THIRTEEN:
DELVING MORE INTO QUALITY ASSESSMENT AND PERFORMANCE IMPROVEMENT ON ESRD

An Overview of the Quality Assessment and Performance Improvement on ESRD

It has been around 40 years since the ESRD program was implemented successfully. Over these long years, the program has successfully provided to more than 400,000 patients with life-saving dialysis therapy. As with any other medical program, each program is subjected to changes keeping in mind the latest innovative scientific findings occurring in the field. This program was no different, as its definitions and demands have been changed. The ever-changing dynamics have spurred calls for advancement in a high-quality program that can address the needs of the changing patient demographics.

However, the call for changes does not in any way undermine the program's credibility as it has for long led to advanced ESRD care that focused at large on improving the technical aspects of care. It had its share of introducing medicines, from erythropoiesis-stimulating agents to active vitamin D for bone disease management.

The program's challenges stem partly from the older and multimorbid patient population that demand urgent attention. Medicare's

Final Rule of the Conditions for Coverage in 2008 has outlined the medical director's role of the dialysis center, by terming the said person as the leader of interdisciplinary team. This same person has been declared responsible for ensuring the highest standards of stringent quality, safety, and care measures offered in the healthcare setting.

The quality assessment and performance improvement process (QAPI) lays overwhelming stress on knowledge and active leadership as the flag bearers of treatment driven by the need to achieve high-quality outcomes in dialysis settings. The program is deemed to be a success as it focuses on adopting a collaborative approach between the director and the dialysis provider. This approach is essential to optimizing the health outcomes of patients by delivering high-quality, evidence-based care.

The ESRD quality incentive program (QIP)

It was in 2011 that the Centers for Medicare & Medicaid Services moved ahead to introduce a pay-for-performance program known to all as the ESRD quality incentive program (QIP). It consisted of yearly varying quality metrics that decide the mechanism of payment reductions that will be suffered by healthcare settings not achieving designated targets during the performance period. Ensuring success in dealing with the QIP necessitates clearly understanding the program's structure, metrics, and scoring methods. Information regarding achievement and nonachievement policies can be accessed publicly through facilities and websites.

By handing over the charge of the leadership role in the quality program of dialysis facilities to the medical director, the top official is entrusted with the responsibility of utilizing all resources and opportunities available to improve patients' lives and induce an actual change in the patient population to facilitate overcoming a dreaded and very challenging chronic disease. The role of the medical director has been summarized in this program which is key to boosting the quality improvement process in the dialysis facility. The associated requirements and programs of QAPI and QIP outline this important role.

All stakeholders from healthcare providers to patients and their families look forward to benefiting from high-quality healthcare. This is because quality is the most focused aspect of any service, but its importance increases to a great extent in a medical setting. This is because, in managing a chronic illness like kidney disease, the care focuses on ensuring all critical issues are addressed to sustain life and avoid death. However, as expected, the definition and the aspects that underline the quality and its measurements vary from organization to organization.

After universal access to dialysis care in the U.S. was implemented around 48 years ago, the medical field has witnessed numerous advances that have altered how ESRD care is provided. Hence, the goal intended as part of this program, which focuses on ensuring rehabilitation to live an active life, has also changed during this period. It has enlarged to a more remarkable program than initially expected and has amassed the latest technologies. This led to home-based therapy initially having a small setting to broaden into a large industry of center-based dialysis care. This has helped pave the way for treating older patients with multiple comorbidities whose population is rising steadily. With time the program has grown and focused on ensuring quality assurance and control.

Role of medical director

The earlier role of the medical director designated for dialysis care was restricted mainly to serving as the physician treating most of the patients in the health care facility. It focused on practicing medicine with every individual patient. However, that was before the expansion of Medicare payments. After the amendments to the Social Security Act in 1973 were passed, the medical director took on the role of a broader care team. This team consisted of nurses, social workers, and dietitians. One of the main points of this Act was that it designated a medical director for each facility as a mandatory practice. This is how the role of the medical director sought to increase the quality outcomes of ESRD patients by putting the medical director in a managerial role.

Medicare ESRD program

Once the Medicare ESRD program was implemented, the rules were explicitly outlined with details of the conditions for coverage (CfC) effective October 2008. The Act put the medical director as the top authority tasked with ensuring all aspects of quality care were delivered in the facility. This marked an increased scope of responsibilities for the medical director.

The tasks assigned to the medical director may be divided into three categories. These included administrative and medical responsibilities, while the third relates to technical insight. This clearly outlines a managerial position that, as per the Centers for Medicare & Medicaid Services (CMS), was enlarged to that of a quarter-full-time position. The responsibilities entailed in the Act are a mammoth task, and the scope of these responsibilities keeps increasing with time as greater challenging clinical situations continue to surface.

The CfC has outlined the duties with which the medical director is entrusted. Apart from the primary role of the medical director stipulates providing leadership for the interdisciplinary team, it also envisions a role catering to individualized patient care and the quality assessment and performance improvement process (QAPI).

Responsibilities of the Medical Director

- Every dialysis facility needs to have a serving Medical Director
- Medical director responsible for the delivery of patient care
- Responsibility includes improving outcomes in the healthcare facility
- Medical Director to be accountable to the governing body
- Other responsibilities also include ensuring the Quality assessment and performance improvement program functions at an optimal level
- Ensuring staff education, training, and performance
- Outlining policies and procedures

QAPI in detail

Led by the medical director, the QAPI consists of an interdisciplinary team of different healthcare workers. Here are the details of the team members:

- Physician (The medical director is mostly entrusted with the overall program in each healthcare setting)
- Registered nurse (the clinical manager mainly)
- Social worker
- Registered dietician

The team is supposed to forge effective communication and allocate the time and attention required to ensure adequate quality assessment while improving performance improvement activities. The goal is positively influence patients' lives by enhancing their health outcomes. The team of QAPI is supposed to meet every month or at least once in three months. The schedule of the meeting depends on state laws governing the facility. All QAPI meetings, activities, and projects under its authority are documented.

There are rules governing the procedure for ensuring quality assessment and performance improvement. As underlined by the program, the following are the parts of the said process:

- Developing, maintaining, implementing, and evaluating an effective quality assessment that is data-driven
- Ensuring an improvement program with all members of the team participating
- The program must function in line with the complexity of the dialysis program and its services
- Focus on indicators that are the hallmark of improved health outcomes
- Focusing on the prevention and reduction of errors related to medical practice
- Maintaining and demonstrating evidence of quality improvement in the dialysis facility
- The dialysis facility must ensure a performance improvement program which the CMS would review

QAPI metrics

This focuses on improving health outcomes and ensuring a reduction in medical errors. For this purpose, indicators or performance measures linked with boosting health outcomes need to be utilized. These indicators are also associated with identifying medical errors and taking steps to reduce them. These include the following:

- Adequacy of dialysis
- Nutritional status
- Mineral metabolism
- Renal bone disease
- Anemia management
- Vascular access
- Medical injuries identification
- Medical errors identification
- Hemodialyzer reuse program in case of reuse of hemodialyzers
- Ensuring patient satisfaction
- Addressing patient grievances
- Maintaining infection control
- Analyzing and documenting infections to record and identify trends
- Establishing baseline information on infection incidence
- Developing recommendations and devising action plans to reduce and minimize infection
- Promoting immunization
- Taking actions to reduce unwanted future incidents

An essential part of the QAPI program is focused on ensuring continued performance improvement monitoring. It also expects the adequate prioritization of improvement activities to be carried out effectively. In recent years, owing to an increased and all-out focus on the efforts emphasizing the target-centered quality and care delivery model based on data, a mindset has emerged that focuses on achieving the target numbers. This trend has become widespread in all dialysis healthcare facilities. In this regard, it is essential to note that though the desire to reach all target metrics will always be welcome and encouraged, it must be remembered that attaining all these goals must align with fulfilling other needs and responsibilities.

This calls for considering the overall situation rather than focusing on one aspect alone.

Considering the broader picture, it becomes apparent that the medical director's leadership role is crucial for the program's success. In hindsight, it is necessary to assisting all dialysis healthcare centers in prioritize improvement projects. It is also required to direct efforts focused on identifying and addressing the systemic issues in the facility. So, to ensure the QAPI program is successful and truly meets all the targets and goals, it is necessary for the true quality issues that harm on many patients to be differentiated from the other aspect that focuses on single-patient outliers. Hence, there is a need to be focused on the entire group of patients. With this in mind, a strategy must be devised that brings about changes that ensure a maximum number of patients can enjoy better care instead of merely focusing on the "outliers." This will contribute to the facility's success and improve patient outcomes. Improving the health outcomes of the patients under care is the program's core. Hence attention must be paid to ensure this across the platform.

Of its intent placed on quality improvement, the program does not focus on solving the issues faced by sick patients who needs to meet the target. The individual patient issue receives attention from direct patient care. The central aspect of quality improvement focuses on the various trends, processes, and infrastructure. It also focuses on access, and adherence to care as being the reason why quality outcomes could not be achieved in a group of patients in a dialysis center. To address all such concerns, the facility needs to be allowed to implement changes based on what benefits the current and future patients. These patients need to be prioritized as they receive care at the center. The QAPI program embodies a process where the medical director moves from a patient care provider role to a role that stipulates population health management.

CHAPTER FOURTEEN:
TRANSFORMING LIVES THROUGH KIDNEY TRANSPLANT

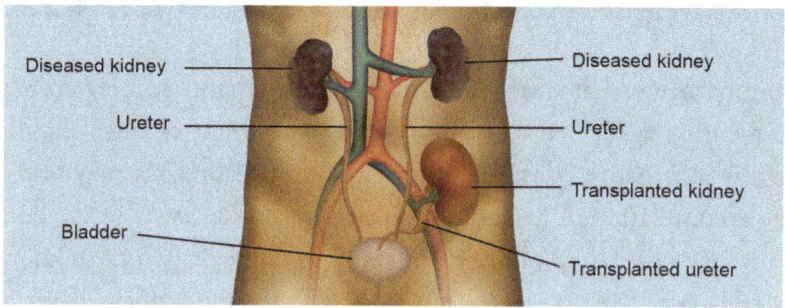

A kidney transplant is carried out to place a healthy kidney inside a person who has suffered from kidney failure. The kidney is placed inside the person whose kidneys have stopped functioning through surgery. The kidney is donated either from a living or a deceased donor. Kidney transplant helps those whose kidneys are no longer functioning to live healthy lives. It allows them to function more or less like normal individuals. Most importantly, it means the person can forego the need to stay on dialysis for a lifetime.

As discussed earlier in the book, the kidneys are two bean-shaped organs in the human body. They are located on each side of the spine and are about the size of a clenched fist. They are found under the abdomen. Kidney filter and remove waste, unwanted minerals, and fluid from the bloodstream via urine.

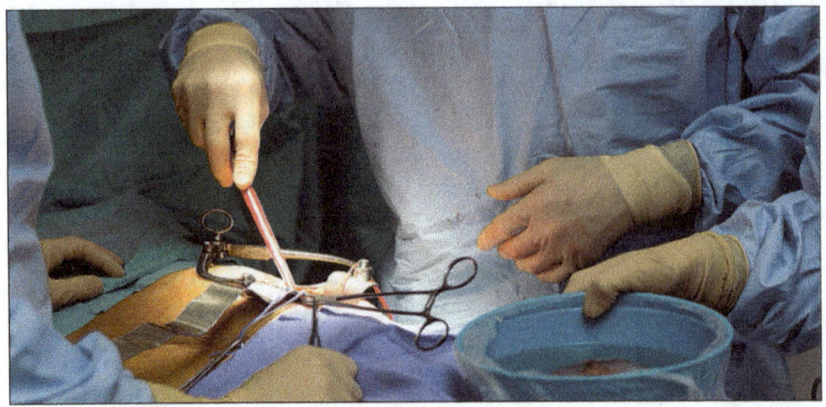

Summarizing what was studied in the earlier chapters, it is pertinent to mention again that when kidneys lose the ability to filter blood, it results in negative consequences for the human body. It may lead to the accumulation of harmful fluid levels and toxic waste in the body. This may raise blood pressure and result in kidney failure, also known as end-stage renal disease. ESRD results once the kidneys have lost about 90% of their ability to function normally. The accumulation of toxins in the body and their fatal effect has already been studied earlier in the book. In such a case, the body slowly drifts towards a shutdown that eventually leads to heart failure and death. Hence, getting treated with an alternative in case of kidney failure is vital to sustain life.

The most common causes of end-stage kidney disease, as discussed earlier are:

- Diabetes
- Uncontrolled high blood pressure persisting for long periods
- Chronic glomerulonephritis (this refers to an inflammation that leads to the scarring of the tiny filters found in the kidneys)
- Polycystic kidney disease

Since it is important for those suffering from end-stage renal disease, to remove waste products from their bloodstream, dialysis or a kidney transplant is imperative to stay alive. Without adhering to one of these alternatives, the person will eventually die.

Why is a kidney transplant necessary?

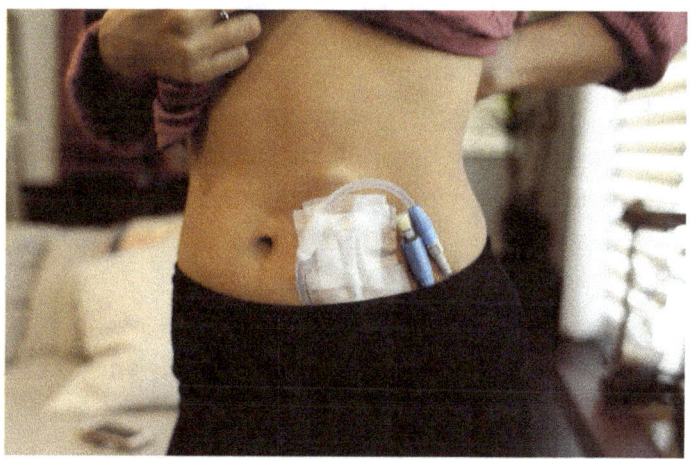

A kidney transplant is one of the treatment options to address the need for filtration following kidney failure. It is a treatment method to sustain life, just like dialysis is required for a lifetime. A kidney transplant helps treat chronic kidney disease or other serious issues like ESRD, allowing kidney recipients to live like ordinary, healthy people can help such kidney recipients live a quality life for a longer time. While dialysis is also used to treat kidney failure, a kidney transplant has many advantages. These include:

- Improved quality of life
- The risk of death is lowered
- Dietary restrictions are less
- Treatment cost is lower

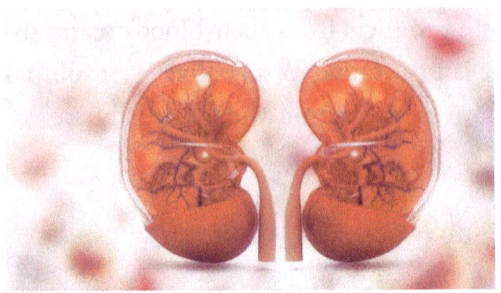

Kidney failure patients can also benefit by receiving a kidney transplant before requiring the need to be on dialysis. This is a procedure called a preemptive kidney transplant. The best part about a kidney transplant is that the recipient no longer needs to stay on dialysis for life. This allows the individual to lead a better life with fewer restrictions.

Since people with kidney failure can live with only one donated kidney in case both kidneys have failed, it paves the way for living-donor kidney transplantation, a worthwhile option to sustain life.

The waiting period for a donor's kidney

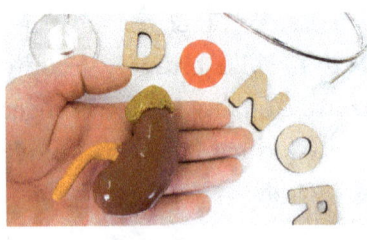

If a compatible living donor isn't found, the person's name will be placed on a kidney transplant waiting list. This means the kidney recipient will be waiting to receive a kidney from a deceased donor.

The duration a person would have to wait for a deceased donor organ depends on many factors. This may be the degree of matching or compatibility between the kidney recipient and the donor. It also depends on the dialysis time and the transplant waitlist. It may also depend on expected survival post-transplant. Sometimes, the person may be lucky to obtain a match within some months, while others would have to wait many years before eventually finding a donor.

The procedure of a kidney transplant

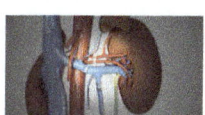

A transplant is scheduled in advance if the kidney recipient receives a kidney from a living donor. Suppose the kidney recipient is being made to wait for a deceased donor. In that case, the kidney recipient must make themselves available immediately by rushing to the hospital when the donor is identified. In such cases, the transplant hospital or institute usually provides kidney recipients and their staff with pagers and cell phones so that it is easy to approach the person and make them available immediately.

After the person arrives at the transplant center, a sample of the kidney recipient's blood is taken for an antibody test. The clearance for surgery is given in case the test result turns out to be a negative crossmatch.

Next, a kidney transplant is carried out under general anesthesia. This process occurs after the person has been given medication to sleep during the surgery. The anesthetic is injected into the body using an intravenous (IV) line in the hand or arm of the kidney recipient.

After the person has fallen asleep, the surgeon makes a cut, known as an incision, in the kidney recipient's abdomen, and then places the donor kidney inside the kidney recipient's body. The arteries and veins coming from the donor's kidney are then connected to the kidney recipient's arteries and veins. Once this process is completed, the blood will flow into the new kidney and throughout the body.

To ensure the kidney recipient can urinate normally, the ureter of the donor kidney placed inside the kidney recipient's body will be attached to the bladder. The ureter is a tube connecting the kidney to the body's bladder.

The kidneys that have ceased to function will be allowed to remain in the body unless they are causing complications. These complications could be high blood pressure or infection.

Aftercare following a transplant

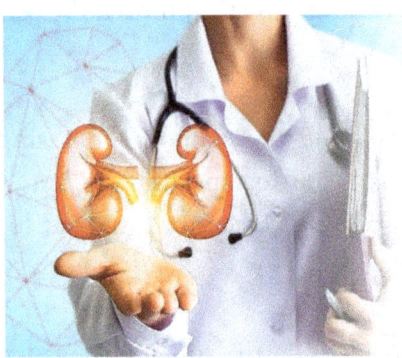

Following the surgery under anesthesia, the person will have the new kidney from the donor put inside their body. The person will then be taken to the recovery room, where they will wake up. The staff will monitor their vital signs until the kidney recipient wakes up and is deemed stable. After that, the individual will be transferred to a hospital room. The person must remain in a hospital in a recovery room for around a week. This stay is necessary even if the kidney recipient feels good after surgery.

How quickly does the new kidney start functioning

The period required for the new kidneys to start functioning as normal kidneys varies from person to person. In some cases, the new kidneys may start clearing waste and extra fluids from the body immediately. However, in some cases, the kidney will start functioning after a few weeks.

It has been observed that a kidney donated by family members has a better chance of working immediately because statistics show that a kidney donated by a family member will usually start working immediately compared to a kidney an unrelated donor has donated. The same is true with a kidney donated by a deceased donor, as it takes time to start functioning normally.

What to expect following a kidney transplant

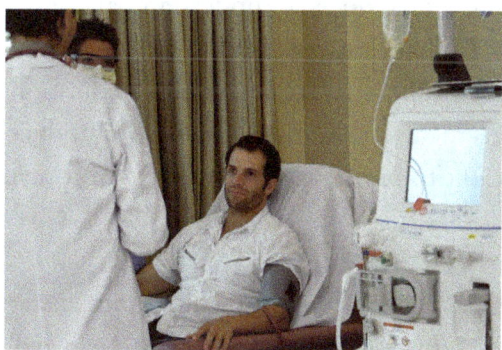

Kidney recipients who have been through the surgery recently may expect to endure pain and soreness in the initial days. This usually happens when the person is healing following the incision required during the transplant. The pain may be significantly felt and occurs at the incision site. Soreness may also accompany pain after the surgery. The person is usually made to stay at the hospital, where the doctor and the healthcare staff monitor the kidney recipient for improvement and note any signs of complications.

Following a transplant, the kidney recipient will also be prescribed a strict schedule of immunosuppressant drugs. This is necessary to prevent the kidney recipient's body from rejecting the new kidney placed inside the body. These kidney recipients will require these drugs every day to ensure their body does not reject the donor's kidney.

What happens after discharge from the hospital

The kidney recipient will usually be discharged from the hospital after one week or a few weeks. However, as a condition of discharge, the doctor needs to inform and educate the person with specific instructions on how and when to take their medications. The person needs to understand these instructions and follow them closely. Suppose the individual does not understand any instructions or has any questions. In that case, they should be asked before discharge so that no mistake occurs in adhering to the medications after leaving the hospital. As mentioned earlier, it is important to continue taking these medications to prevent the body from rejecting the new donor kidney.

The medications are only one of the aspects necessary aspects that must to be kept in mind. The kidney recipient will also need to discuss with the doctor a checkup schedule that would need to be followed after the surgery and even after discharge from the hospital.

Once the person has been discharged, they must keep regular appointments with the doctor and the transplant team. These appointments are necessary to ensure that the kidney is functioning optimally. The purpose of the appointment is to evaluate how well the kidney is functioning.

It is important to mention again that the person will need to take the immunosuppressant drugs as prescribed by the doctor. Apart from these drugs, the person may be prescribed additional necessary drugs that are necessary to prevent the risk of contracting the infection. The person will also have to be vigilant by monitoring their body for warning signs that suggest their body has rejected the new kidney. The possible warning signs are swelling, pain, swelling, and flu-like symptoms.

The total time to recover may last up to six months. Following up regularly with the doctor is extremely important, at least for the first two months.

Benefits of a kidney transplant

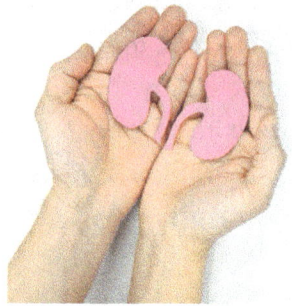

There are many benefits of opting for a kidney transplant. Experts often term a kidney transplant as the best option for people diagnosed with long-term kidney ailments. This option has many benefits over dialysis.

Some of the important benefits are discussed below.

Dialysis is no longer required

Dialysis is life-saving for an individual with ESRD. A person whose kidneys have ceased to function normally undoubtedly requires dialysis without which they cannot survive. However, dialysis has its cons, such as being very time-consuming and accompanied by different issues that may shorten life expectancy. Besides, the risk of infection is very high among dialysis patients.

This is where a kidney transplant comes to the rescue. A kidney transplant means that the patient will no longer need to stay on dialysis. People with kidney transplants also have an advantage over dialysis patients because they usually live longer. They also enjoy a better quality of life as compared to dialysis patients.

A kidney transplant allows a person more energy for daily activities

It has been observed that people who undergo a kidney transplant feel more energetic. It allows them to cater to their daily life routines in a better way. It gives them more energy for other activities, like travel, work, and going out. Those with a kidney transplant can even go on a holiday as it is easier this way. A kidney transplant also allows one to exercise and even engage in sports.

Carrying out these activities while being on dialysis takes work. On dialysis, even minor physical exertions that were previously easy to perform will become difficult after being put on dialysis.

Reductions in dietary restrictions

This is one main benefit of undergoing a kidney transplant. The majority of the patients on dialysis will need to follow a strict dietary regimen. They will need to abstain from consuming certain foods. The intake of fluids will also need to be restricted. In contrast, people who underwent a kidney transplant will have far fewer restrictions imposed on them. They will have greater freedom to eat and drink than to dialysis patients.

Improvement in sex life and fertility

Following a kidney transplant, the sex life and fertility of a person improve to a great extent as compared to a patient who stays on dialysis. Following a transplant, a woman of childbearing age can conceive.

However, in some cases, the transplant team may ask the woman to wait a year before conceiving a baby. Overall, the sex life and fertility of a kidney transplant patient improve as compared to a patient put on dialysis.

Kidney transplant outlook in the U.S.

The survival rates of those diagnosed with long-term kidney disease in the U.S. continue to improve. The last three decades have witnessed continuous improvements. However, there is still room available for further improvement. These outcomes can be improved, and the future will hold better news for those with ailing kidney conditions.

Experts voice their support for kidney transplants in the presence of available research and studies. Experts and other professionals term a kidney transplant a better means for most patients suffering from end-stage kidney disease based on the statistics available. According to experts and the transplant team, this option is far better than being made to live a lifetime on dialysis. Although some kidney grafts will eventually fail in the future, methods are available to prolong the survival time of these grafts, leading to an improved lifespan of the patients. This not only further boosts the quality of life of these patients but also translates into a lesser burden on the healthcare sector. It also serves as a light at the end of the tunnel since it means more kidneys will be available for the 90,000 people waiting for a transplant nationwide.

Since the mid-1990s, improvement has been witnessed steadily in kidney transplant survival rates. This fact holds true for both the patients and the kidney graft. The good news is that these positive outcomes have been witnessed despite the general population's steep rise in risk factors, such as diabetes, obesity, and other related conditions.

These positive trends have been identified by healthcare organizations in the U.S. They serve as a positive reminder that opportunities are available to improve kidney transplant survival in the country further.

It is important to note that kidney transplantation involves grafting a healthy kidney into a recipient after ensuring the deceased or living donor has been screened to ensure compatibility with the recipient. Since the threat of the body rejecting the new kidney always persists, the patients are put on immunosuppressive drugs for a lifetime. The good news is that the long-term survival of kidney grafts has shown positive results.

The following five-year survival rate table demonstrates how kidney transplant survival rates have improved in the U.S. since the mid-1990s.

	Deceased donors	Living donors
1996–1999	66.2%	79.5%
2012–2015	78.2%	88.1%

CHAPTER FIFTEEN:
BENEFITS OF MEDICARE COVERAGE FOR END STAGE RENAL DISEASE (ESRD) PEOPLE

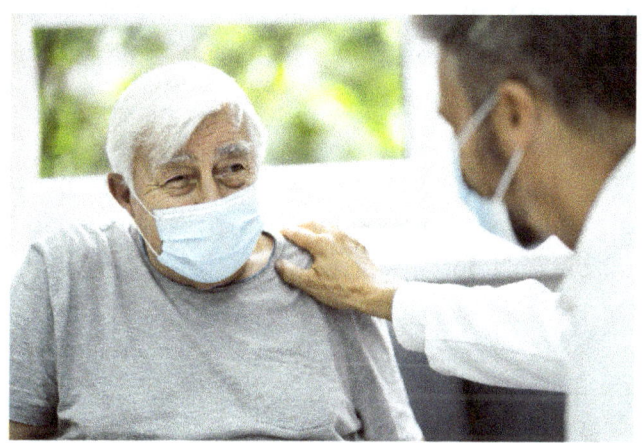

Numerous programs have been aimed at saving and improving the lives of Americans suffering from different ailments, especially at the federal level. However, the Medicare end-stage renal disease program initiated in 1973 has allowed more than 1 million Americans to benefit from life-saving renal replacement therapy. This program has marked an unprecedented move that became the reason for the survival of around a million people, most of whom would have died. The program came into being because of the Social Security Amendments of 1972. Before this program commenced, the situation could have been more promising for kidney patients as treatment was marred due to the high costs associated with such treatment and the limited number of dialysis machines. Before the commencement of this program in 1972, hospitals had formed special committees to decide who would receive dialysis treatment owing to the limited resources and finances, while the others could not possibly receive the treatment and were left to die.

However, things have changed, and now every American citizen is eligible for Medicare benefits if diagnosed with End-Stage Renal Disease (ESRD) disease. Unlike other treatment programs, there is no age limit for such individuals. Patients with ESRD are eligible for the program even if they are under 65. Under this program, Medicare will cover the medical expenses associated with treating late-stage kidney disease.

Since ESRD is an advanced chronic disease marked by permanent kidney failure, an individual's kidneys have failed to function, leaving them with the only options of long-term dialysis or a kidney transplant to survive. Now all those diagnosed with ESRD can qualify for Medicare coverage regardless of age. This means a person would be eligible for the program under 65.

End-Stage Renal Disease Treatment Choice (ETC) model

This model came to the fore after being finalized by the Centers for Medicare and Medicaid Services (CMS) in 2020. The program has improved healthcare access for all those diagnosed with ESRD. Before the enactment of this model, some individuals had lost coverage for these services or were required to pay additional insurance premiums.

This treatment model has revolutionized renal care by protecting to kidney patients from losing health coverage or overpaying for it. It allows them to receive life-saving treatments. Medicare coverage may vary depending on whether an individual is insured by group health or Medicare.

ESRD patient and private insurance and group coverage

As part of the ETC model, group health plan providers are forbidden from differentiating or limiting benefits or terminating coverage. Furthermore, they are also forbidden from raising premium prices for patients who have an ESRD diagnosis.

Patients with the group health plan coverage must enroll in Medicare within 30 months following an ESRD diagnosis. This period is referred to as the coordination period. Based on the 30-month timeframe, private insurance and Medicare work together but in different ways.

During the first 30 month, when an ESRD patient is on health services, the group health insurance is liable to pay first in the healthcare costs incurred while Medicare would act as the secondary payer for the remainder of the costs. These payments will be made for Medicare-approved services.

This mode of payment and responsibility switches after 30 months. Now Medicare would pay first, while the group health plan would cover the remaining costs.

After an ESRD patient has enrolled in Medicare and for the 30 months coordination period, the benefits will be applicable at different times depending on whether the patient receives dialysis service or a kidney transplant.

Dialysis Treatment and Medicare

Following an ESRD patient's treatment with dialysis, Medicare benefits will be offered during the fourth month of the treatment. The treatment will be offered in a Medicare-approved dialysis center. However, if ESRD patients learn how to administer the dialysis treatment at home, they will be eligible for Medicare benefits earlier. In some cases, the treatment costs as early as the first month of dialysis will be covered by Medicare. These include circumstances when an ESRD patient undergoes and completes a training program from a Medicare-approved facility on home dialysis or commences a home dialysis training program expected to be completed soon. These benefits will also apply if the patient gives self-dialysis treatment during the first three months.

The ESRD patients on dialysis treatment will continue receiving Medicare benefits for 12 months following the last month of dialysis treatment.

Kidney transplant and Medicare

An ESRD patient admitted to a Medicare-approved facility or hospital for a kidney transplant or any other transplant-related services required for preparing for a transplant within two months will be eligible to receive Medicare benefits within the same month. The transplant recipients can benefit from Medicare until 36 months after kidney transplants.

These patients also benefit from requaring for Medicare under the ETC model if additional dialysis or a transplant is required later. In the following case, the coordination period spanning 30 months will apply.

Services covered by Medicare

ESRD patients usually require long-term dialysis or a kidney transplant. However, Medicare covers other services, too, apart from these two key services for the affected persons. If a patient is eligible for Medicare benefits due to an ESRD diagnosis, Medicare will cover all the necessary medical services, not those related to ESRD.

Medicare would be paying only for the approved services in all cases. This means that Medicare coverage will not be included for prescription drugs. To enjoy prescription drug coverage, patients with ESRD will have to look for another source. This could be primary insurance, a drug plan, creditable coverage, or a Medicare Advantage Prescription Drug plan.

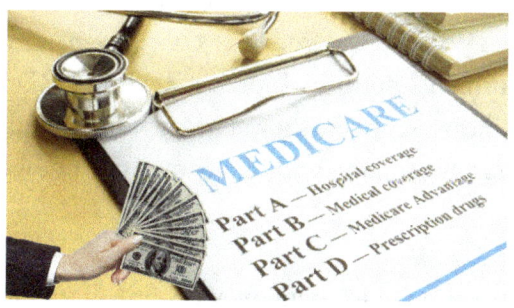

Medicare's special plans

ESRD is a complex medical condition that needs many resources. For treating patients with ESRD, specialized coverage is essential. The good news is that Medicare Advantage covers these needs through special needs plans. Since it is established that there are only a few other pre-existing conditions that happen to be more complex than ESRD, intensive care for ESRD outweighs the costs for many other diseases. The specific plans provided under the Medicare Advantage System are a light at the end of the tunnel for ESRD patients. All these plans are designed to assist patients with special needs, including ESRD.

Conditions on which the coverage would end, continue or resume

Medicare coverage will end if individual benefits from Medicare only because of ESRD 12 months after they have stopped dialysis. It will also end 36 months after a kidney transplant has been completed and the person no longer requires dialysis.

The Medicare coverage for a patient with ESRD will continue in case dialysis is restarted within 12 months after the time dialysis was stopped. The coverage will also continue in case of a kidney transplant within 12 months. Individual with ESRD can also benefit from Medicare services, they start or resume dialysis or go for another kidney transplant within 36 months following a kidney transplant.

The Medicare coverage for patients with ESRD will resume in case the ESRD Medicare ends and the patient resumes dialysis or goes for the option of getting another kidney transplant for kidney failure. In this case, the mediocre coverage will start immediately without the need to wait for any time.

Eligibility criteria for Medicare if a patient has ESRD

In case an individual has been diagnosed with ESRD, then regardless of age, Medicare can be received under the following conditions:

- If the individual's kidneys no longer work
- Regular dialysis is required
- If the individual has had a kidney transplant
- If the individual has fulfilled the required amount of time under Social Security or as a government employee or the Railroad Retirement Board (RRB)
- Individuals who are already availing or are eligible for Social Security and Railroad Retirement benefits
- If the individual is a spouse or a dependent of the person who fulfills the conditions above

ESRD Patients and Medicare Advantage

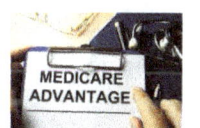

Medicare Advantage, or MA, is an option for those on Medicare coverage diagnosed with ESRD. The Medicare Advantage is also called Medicare Part C. It is a broad program that works as an all-in-one health insurance plan. It is unique in the sense that it offers the combined benefits of Medicare Parts A, B, and at times D, making it one convenient plan.

There are numerous benefits to opting for Medicare Advantage. Firstly, ESRD patients, by availing of this plan, will only have to pay attention to one plan to manage their needs. It also means there will be only one insurance card to address their needs.

Secondly, some plans will bear costs equal to or even lower than Medicare. The premiums may be as low as 0 dollars.

Thirdly, many plans will include extra benefits, like dental, vision, and hearing.

Fourthly, ESRD patients, can save on prescription costs, such as kidney medications and insulin by availing of this plan.

Fifthly, spending will be limited as annual out-of-pocket costs have been capped.

Medicare Advantage compared to other Medicare plans

As mentioned above, Medicare Advantage replaces Medicare Parts A, B, and C. Comparing the costs, benefits, and potential to save money makes this plan a good choice for those diagnosed with ESRD.

When an ESRD patient selects a Medicare Advantage plan and prescription coverage, it implies that the patient will be fully insured. Hence, a separate prescription plan will not be required that has its premium. This will allow the individual with an ESRD diagnosis to save money while benefiting from health care.

Medicare Advantage also offers benefits to patients diagnosed with ESRD that will not be available in the case of traditional Medicare. These benefits will include different facilities, such as those related to dental, vision, hearing care, and transportation.

An significant difference between Medicare Advantage plans and traditional Medicare plans is that private health insurance companies manage the former while the federal government manage the latter.

Choosing between Medicare Advantage plans and traditional Medicare plans

Another important benefit for patients with ESRD is that the Medicare Advantage plans utilize networks, such as employer group health plans. This will allow these individuals to opt for in-network doctors and avoid extra costs.

Summarizing the benefits of Medicare Advantage plans, patients diagnosed with ESRD can benefit from better coverage. These plans also allow them to benefit from lower premium costs, allowing them to save money. It also offers the convenience of being an all-in-one plan, allowing individuals to avoid doing the extra work required to benefit from the same umbrella of services through different plans. Though it is always necessary to consider all the costs when determining which health plan bests suits an individual, the Medicare Advantage plans are the most convenient option for patients with an ESRD diagnosis.

It is important to note that an ESRD patient will not need supplemental insurance with Medicare Advantage. This is because the total coverage will be included with Medicare Advantage plan, such as prescription coverage. Since all of the patient's coverage is included in a single plan, supplemental coverage will not be required. The individual will be considered fully insured. Hence, purchasing a separate prescription drug plan will not be needed. This also means no Medicare Supplement plan will be required since the individual will enjoy all their coverage benefits in 1 plan. This will allow them to forego the need to opt for several programs as they can benefit from one insurance card.

CHAPTER SIXTEEN:
HEALTHY LIFESTYLE

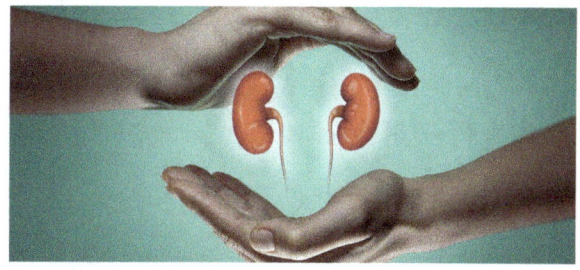

The kidneys are important organs about the fist size located at the bottom of the rib cage. Found on both sides of the spine, the kidneys perform several essential functions critical to sustaining life. Among the many vital functions of the kidney, they filter the bloodstream by eliminating excess water, waste products, and other impurities via urine through the bladder. Besides this critical function, the kidneys regulate pH, salt, and potassium. They also help regulate blood pressure through the secretion of hormones and play their role in controlling red blood cell production.

The kidneys have other important roles as well. They activate a form of vitamin D required to help the body absorb calcium. This is necessary for building bones and also to regulate muscle function.

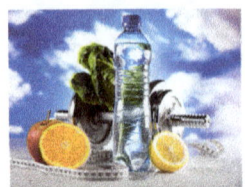

Hence, owing to the many important functions of kidneys, it is imperative to maintain kidney health. This is critical to your overall health. Healthy kidneys help the body filter and expel waste adequately. Without removing these waste products, the human body's survival will be at risk. Besides, the hormones required to help the body function properly will only be produced with healthy kidneys.

Importance of preventing chronic kidney disease and the risk factors

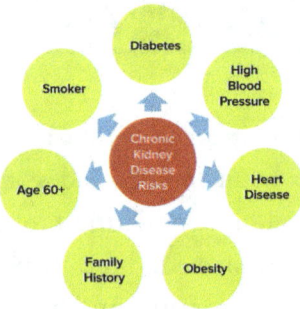

Many risk factors increase the chances of contracting chronic kidney disease. People with a few conditions are more likely to develop kidney disease. These risk factors include the following:

- Diabetes
- High blood pressure
- Heart disease
- Family history of kidney failure

Your risk is considerably increased if you have any of the above conditions.

Ways to keep your kidneys healthy

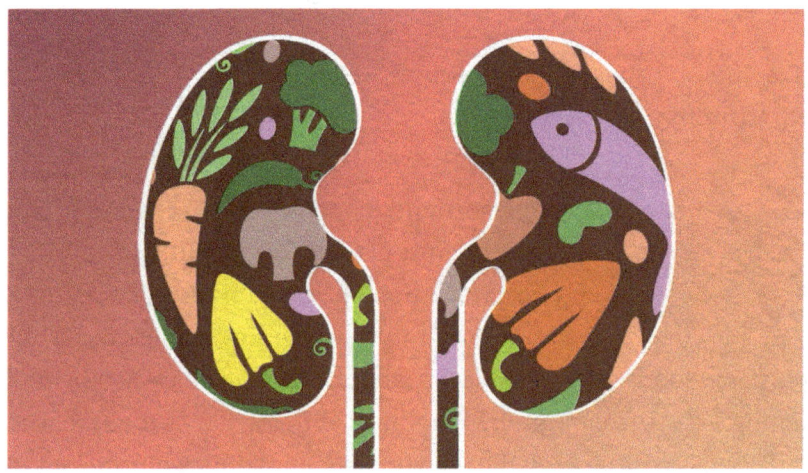

The health of the kidneys can be maintained, and damage can be avoided by preventing and managing health conditions that are the reason behind causing damage to the kidneys. These include conditions like diabetes and high blood pressure. Here are a few steps that can be taken to ensure your whole body remains healthy and functions optimally, including the kidneys.

Whenever you visit for a medical checkup, you need to ask your healthcare provider to look into your kidneys' health. The problem is that kidney disease in the early stages shows no signs or symptoms. The only way to detect early kidney damage is to get tested. This will help you find out about your kidney health. Following a kidney test, the doctor will be able to identify how often you need to get tested to determine your kidney health. This will ensure you can keep your kidneys healthy and address any problems that may spiral out of control.

A kidney test will also help determine if you have developed any problem, such as a urinary tract infection (UTI). Such conditions can cause kidney damage if it is not treated.

Healthy food intake

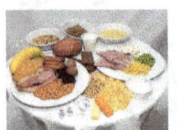

Selecting the right foods to eat is very important. Following the proper diet can help improve and maintain overall body health. You must select foods that are healthy for the body and the heart. For this purpose, foods like fresh fruits and fresh vegetables are helpful. Eating a diet of whole grains combined with low-fat or foods that are fat-free dairy products will help you maintain kidney health. Always consume healthy meals, and eliminate salt and added sugars from your diet. The sodium intake must be reduced to less than 2,300 milligrams each day. Try to limit the intake of added sugars in your body. Added sugars must be less than 10 percent of your daily calories intake.

How to make healthy food choices

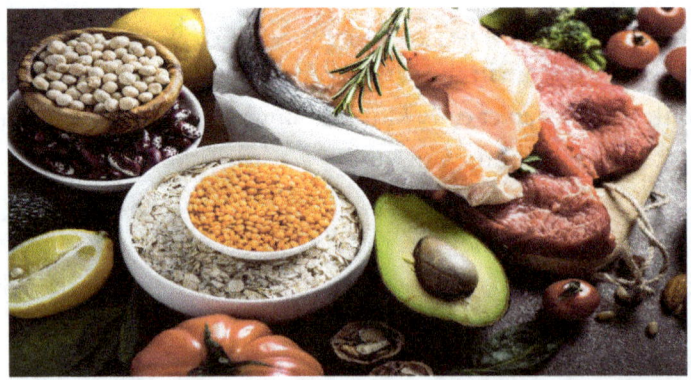

There are many tips for making healthy food choices. You can start by cooking food with a mix of spices and replacing them with salt. Veggie toppings should be selected that are beneficial to your health. Examples include broccoli. For pizza, you may use peppers. Try using more baked products instead of frying food, like boiling meat, chicken, and fish. Fried foods must be avoided. Foods without gravy must be consumed. Try avoiding added fats in your diet. The same applies to added sugars. Select food that contains little or no added sugars at all. It would help to reduce whole milk intake and replace it with 2 percent milk. Finally, you must drink and cook with fat-free milk, also known as skim milk. You may use low-fat milk and milk products in place.

Eating foods that are made up of whole grains is important. These include whole wheat, brown rice, oats, and whole-grain corn. They must be a part of your daily diet. For enjoying toast and sandwiches you can use whole-grain bread. Try substituting brown rice with white rice. This should be the course for home-cooked meals and when you are dining out.

A good idea is to always read food labels before buying them. This will allow you to make informed choices. It will give you a clear idea of selecting foods low in saturated fats, trans fats, salt, added sugars and cholesterol. All such precautions will help you maintain your overall health and prevent the rise of any problem that threatens the health of your kidneys. You need to take steps to slow down his habit when consuming snacks. An example is to reduce the quantity of food that is high in calories and replace them with food that is low in calories. You can start by eating a bag of low-fat popcorn instead of high-calorie food like a cake. Another example is to peel an orange and consume it instead of drinking orange juice. This way, you can cut down the calorie intake considerably.

Also, maintaining a written record of your food will help serve the purpose. Such a habit is crucial in helping avoid overeating or eating foods high in fat or calories.

Research has concluded that following a diet plan based on healthy foods, such as the ones mentioned above, helps you maintain your blood pressure at normal levels. If you are already faced with high blood pressure or other problems that are harmful to the kidneys, such as diabetes or heart disease, then you need to consult a dietitian and follow their advice closely. Regular physical activity must be a part of your daily routine.

Try being active for at least 30 minutes or more than that almost every day. If you do not engage in activities that require you to be active, consult with a healthcare provider immediately about how to adapt to lead an active physical life. This will help you determine the physical activity you can engage in to boost your body's health. The right tips from a professional will help you start a physically active schedule that will benefit your health.

Always maintain a healthy weight

Maintaining a healthy weight is important for your health and kidneys. Obesity or weight gain brings in many issues and also harms your kidneys. If you are obese or overweight, start working immediately to reduce weight. Working with a health care provider or even a dietitian is necessary in such a case to create a realistic weight-loss plan and implement it. It is time to look into weight control and physical activity resources to ensure you start losing weight and maintain healthy body weight.

Sleep enough

Getting an adequate amount of sleep is essential for health. In this regard, experts suggest aiming for 7 to 8 hours of sound sleep every day. It lowers stress levels and helps in keeping you fresh throughout the day. If you are having difficulty sleeping, start taking steps to ensure you can enjoy 8 hours of sound sleep every day.

Quit smoking

Smoking or using tobacco in any other way is harmful to health. If you are already addicted to this habit, seek professional help to get rid of this habit. Using tobacco in any form harms your health, including the kidneys.

Limit alcohol intake

Drinking too much alcohol is harmful to your health. It causes an increase in blood pressure besides adding extra calories that contribute to weight gain. If you drink alcohol regularly, then try limiting its intake.

Engage in stress-reducing activities

Learning ways to manage stress is essential. Try learning professionally recommended ways to relax and cope with problems that are causing stress. This will help you improve your emotional and physical health. Physical activity has the potential to help reduce stress. Mind and body practices also serve the same purpose,

Managing key risk factors, such as diabetes, high blood pressure, and heart disease

If you have any of these three problems, you need to keep them in control to maintain the health of your kidneys. Diabetes, high blood pressure, or heart disease are known to cause damage to the kidneys. The best way to protect against kidney damage is to control these risk factors. You can start by keeping blood glucose levels at a healthy level. You need to check your blood glucose levels, also known as blood sugar levels. This is a crucial way to manage your diabetes. Your doctor could recommend testing your blood glucose levels more than once daily.

Also, maintaining normal blood pressure is important. The blood pressure levels for people with diabetes should be below 140/90 mm Hg. In case you have high blood pressure, then consult with a doctor. It would help if you focused more on your diet or may even require medications to keep it under control. It is important to take all your medicines as prescribed by the doctor. You can also discuss taking certain blood pressure medicines, called ACE inhibitors and ARBs, with your doctor. These medicines will help protect your kidneys.

Precaution must also be exercised regarding the daily use of over-the-counter pain medications. Using nonsteroidal anti-inflammatory drugs (NSAIDs) regularly can cause damage to your health, especially the kidneys. An example is ibuprofen.

You also need to decrease the risk of heart attacks and stroke. For this purpose, you need to keep your cholesterol levels in check. Two types of cholesterol are found in your blood: LDL and HDL. The former is known as "bad" cholesterol. It can build up in the bloodstream and lead to the clogging of your blood vessels. This may lead to a heart attack or stroke. The latter is known as "good" cholesterol as it helps remove the "bad" cholesterol from the bloodstream. You would need to undergo a cholesterol test as it will also help measure another type of blood fat called triglycerides.

The important tasks of Healthy Kidneys at a glance:

- Regulating the fluid levels of your body
- Filtering wastes and toxins from the bloodstream
- Releasing a hormone responsible for regulating blood pressure
- Activating vitamin D to ensure the maintenance of healthy bones
- Releasing hormone involved in the production of red blood cells
- Keeping blood minerals in balance (examples are sodium, phosphorus, and potassium)

Examples of problems caused by kidney disease:

- Heart disease
- Stroke
- Heart attack
- High blood pressure
- Weak bones
- Nerve damage (neuropathy)
- Kidney failure
- End-stage kidney disease (ESRD)
- Anemia or low red blood cell count

Assessing your risk for kidney disease

There are five main risk factors for kidney disease. Controlling them will help reduce the threat of suffering from kidney disease. These are:

- Diabetes
- High blood pressure
- Heart disease
- Family history of kidney failure or problems mentioned above
- Obesity

Some additional risk factors need to be kept in mind, they are:

- Being aged 60 or above
- Low birth weight
- Prolonged use of NSAIDs (type of painkillers, examples are ibuprofen and naproxen)
- Lupus
- Autoimmune disorders
- Chronic urinary tract infections
- Kidney stones

Learning about these risk factors will make you aware of kidney health. It is a step towards leading a healthier life. This way you will have an understanding of where you stand.

Recognizing the symptoms of kidney problem

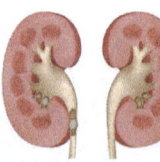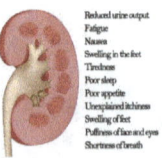

Reduced urine output
Fatigue
Nausea
Swelling in the feet
Tiredness
Poor sleep
Poor appetite
Unexplained itchiness
Swelling of feet
Puffiness of face and eyes
Shortness of breath

Many signs suggest trouble. However, the majority of the people suffering from early kidney disease demonstrate no symptoms. This means detecting early symptoms is critical. The problem is that kidney disease may have advanced once the symptoms appear. You need to pay attention to these symptoms closely:

- Fatigue
- Weakness
- Difficulty urinating
- Blood urine with urine turning pink or dark
- Foamy urine
- Increased need to urinate (especially at night)
- Increased thirst
- Puffy eyes
- Swelling in face, hands, abdomen

Getting tested is important – here is how

If you or your loved one fall under the category of those at high risk for kidney disease, immediately discuss this with a primary-care physician, including the tests required to determine the risk. Your doctor may order other tests as well to determine the risk and how much damage has been caused to your kidneys,

Here are three life-saving tests.

Blood Pressure test

High blood pressure harms your body by damaging the small blood vessels, known as glomeruli, in the kidneys. As discussed earlier in the book, these are small filtering units. This significantly damages your kidney. It is also the second primary reason for kidney failure after diabetes.

BP of 140/90 is deemed good for most people. BP below 130/80 is judged better if you have chronic kidney disease. A BP below 120/80 will be considered best. You must check with your doctor about the values that are best.

Urine test

This test allows traces of a protein called albumin to be detected in the urine. Albuminuria as it is known, could be an early sign of kidney disease. If regular amounts of albumin and other proteins are found in the urine, a condition known as proteinuria would indicate kidney damage.

If the test shows an amount measuring less than 30 mg of albumin per gram of urinary creatinine, it is a good count. Creatinine is a regular waste product.

Glomerular Filtration Rate (GFR)

This test allows the doctor to measure how well your kidneys perform when blood filtering. Doctors can calculate the glomerular filtration rate (GFR) by measuring blood creatinine levels.

A score of over 90 is generally considered suitable.. If the score is 60-89, it should be monitored. A score of less than 60, consistent for three months, indicates kidney disease.

Staying Healthy

A few steps are a must for those with kidney disease. These are:

- Maintaining lower high blood pressure
- Managing blood sugar levels
- Avoiding NSAIDs
- Reducing salt intake
- Keeping protein consumption in moderate quantities
- Going for an annual flu shot

Important steps to follow for maintaining good kidney health

Exercising regularly, controlling weight, following a balanced diet, quitting smoking, quitting alcohol, staying hydrated, monitoring cholesterol levels, getting an annual physical checkup, and learning about your family medical history will help you maintain your overall kidney health and keep them in good shape.

Important fact about the U.S.

Around 1 in 10 Americans who are aged 20 or above demonstrate evidence of kidney disease. The bad news is that some forms of kidney disease prevalent in the U.S. are progressive. It implies that in such cases, the disease gets worse as time passes. Kidneys eventually fail once they are no longer functioning to the extent of removing waste from the bloodstream.

CHAPTER SEVENTEEN:
HOW TO BECOME AN EFFECTIVE NURSE

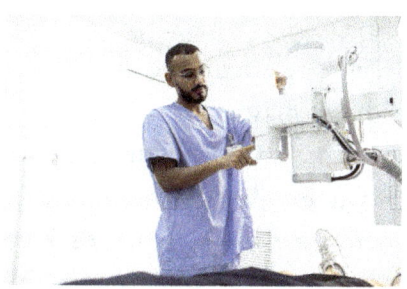

Nurses play a vital role in any healthcare system. Being an effective nurse requires much more than just a degree. Being one of the most challenging professional careers, nursing requires many skills to be successful. It is not just a straightforward career path. The role of nursing envisions a lot more than just a high level of education. It mandates a strong sense of dedication to dispense the key responsibilities. Furthermore, physical and mental endurance must be effective at a nursing job. The world outside the nursing school is quite vast, and nurses must equip themselves with some specific personality traits and skillset to improve the health outcomes of the patients.

To be influential nurses, along with the top skills, nurses need to be resilient against stress. Here are some of the qualities that good nurses must embody.

Good organizational behavior is key to the successful dispensation of nursing responsibilities

Experts often cite organization as the essential trait a nurse must demonstrate through their behavior. The medical field has many ups and downs. From a chaotic shift to a patient's health spiraling out of control, nurses must be organized to adapt to the testing times and prioritize what is best for the patients.

Nurses have many vital roles to play, and organization becomes a critical skill nurses must master to make their job easier and positively impact the patients and the entire healthcare team. The importance of this trait cannot be underestimated because it is critical to keeping the patients safe and ensuring they are healing. Besides, organizational skills are required to keep a close eye on everything that is going on about the patients.

Being multitasking and organized is essential to be a practical nurse. From noticing the small and minor details about the patient to collecting labs and ensuring patients take medications on time, all the tasks regarding a patient's health need to be prioritized and organized.

Critical thinking is essential to come up with effective solutions to healthcare challenges

Once again, this is another important skill required to be effective in a healthcare setting. The ability to think logically, clearly, and intellectually is the key to successfully dispensing the responsibilities and tasks assigned to a nurse. This also is one of the nurses' highly demanded skills because, just like good organization, this key is critical to ensuring improved patient outcomes. Since it directly impacts patient care and affects health outcomes, critical thinking is essential for offering self-sufficiency to nurses.

Critical thinking is a trait that instills in nurses an ability to logically and critically analyze facts and challenges to find a lasting solution. A lack of critical thinking implies that the nurses would fail to reach objective conclusions. This will make them continuously struggle throughout their careers.

To elucidate the importance of critical thinking, consider, for example, the case of forensic nursing. This career, by all standards, is a very lucrative one but one that comes with numerous challenges. Such a job setting requires an eye for detail and an in-depth insight into rational thinking. Though it offers numerous benefits and lucrative salaries, nurses can only be effective in this role if they fail to participate in evidence-gathering procedures. This failure would be evident in case they cannot think critically. Most importantly, nurses must be able to interpret, evaluate and analyze the facts. The same is true for other fields of nursing that make it necessary for nurses to practice critical thinking and undergo a continuous learning process.

Good communication skills are critical to improved healthcare

If one skill is mandatory in the nursing profession, by all means, it is effective communication skills. Lacking this crucial skill means a nurse would fail to contribute to their role effectively. The importance of good communication skills cannot be denied. This is because lacking this critical skill would put patient's lives at risk.

The role of a nurse requires them to go through much data that needs to be collected and conveyed to the relevant healthcare givers.

There is no room for errors in the collection and handling of essential data related to the patients. The data needs to be interpreted as accurately as possible. Just imagine a scenario where a nurse misses patient information or hears the wrong orders. Just think about any misinformation on the part of the nurse. All these mistakes will endanger the life of the patient. A nurse needs to take instructions from coworkers and supervisors. Any minor hurdle in communication will lead to a problematic situation, especially in high-pressure situations.

Hence, impeccable verbal and non-verbal techniques are essential in a nursing role. It becomes all the more critical when it comes to listening, tracking, and presenting the information related to a patient. Besides verbal and nonverbal skills, nurses must stay updated with the latest technological tools, such as healthcare software. This is necessary to facilitate information transfer to the relevant persons. Besides, good communication skills are necessary to address the communication barriers between them and the patients or their families. Proactive communication is also important, as patients are usually anxious about their health. They must be provided with precise and reliable information about their health and treatment. From test results to diagnosis and treatment plans, every aspect of information needs to be conveyed explicitly without any vagueness.

How can nurses improve their skills to play a more effective role?

With the advancement in medical knowledge, professional development has become the key to nursing success. With jobs in the nursing sector continuing to grow, professional development has become increasingly important. At the national level, the jobs for registered nurses have recorded a steep rise. Over the next decade, jobs in this sector are projected to grow by nine percent. The U.S. Bureau of Labor Statistics has provided this figure.

Back in 2020, nurses held around 3.1 million jobs, with around 60% employed in hospital settings, while the rest were employed in home healthcare services, nursing facilities, physicians' offices, clinics, schools, the military, and other places.

Since the nursing sector will likely grow in the coming years, the critical question is how nurses can improve their nursing skills. Here are a few tips to get started.

Do not stop the learning process

Nurses with a BSN or a bachelor's degree in nursing have come a long way. They are equipped with the skill set required to grow and ensure the complete delivery of safe patient care. However, the learning process must not end. If studying for an additional degree impossible, then a nurse must use other educational opportunities. These could be activities like studying for a certification or volunteering for different causes to enhance experience-based learning. At times, simply attending workshops help improve the critical skills a nurse requires. Examples of suitable certifications, such as licensed nursing assistants, can be acquired.

Boosting skills to communicate effectively

The importance of good communication skills has already been discussed above. However, improving this key skill set, requires a lot of practice, time, and effort, in the long run. The importance of acquiring and enhancing this critical skill must be recognized as it is the key to providing quality healthcare to patients.

The key to the successful delivery of services is based on the ability to be a good listener. This requires an attentive role and the ability not to be distracted in the heat of the moment. A feeling of distraction or rush makes nursing tasks challenging to manage and sends a negative message to patients and their families.

When trying to boost this primary skill, nurses need to adopt a proactive approach where they learn to be good listeners and can convey information based on the patient's perspective. This is because a nurse's role also encompasses educating and counseling the patients from their perspective. In this regard, learning to communicate with patients based on their culture, opinions, and concerns is necessary.

Learn to adopt a patient-centric approach

At the heart of healthcare services lies the philosophy of adopting a patient-centric approach and focusing on the people. Since the nurses have to be multitasked and are deeply involved with their responsibilities, it is expected that nurses may need to catch up on their fundamental responsibility of interacting with their patients.

The quality that a nurse must learn over time is to connect with people. The ability to give undivided attention to the patients makes the difference. The main skill that must be learned is always to focus on maintaining and staying attentive to the patients and about ways to improve their lives.

CHAPTER EIGHTEEN:
LIFE STORIES OF AN R.N. TREATING DIALYSIS PATIENT

Starting as a registered nurse, I have acquired immense experience in the field of dialysis, especially the various technicities surrounding the treatment protocol and its practical implementation. I found my inspiration and desire to serve in this field because of the early family experiences that shaped my attitude toward kidney disease and its treatment. As a young lady, I spent much of my early years living with my grandparents. Since my parents were working abroad and I had to stay behind to complete my education, my grandparents, who lived with me, were an integral part of my life. However, much to my dismay, I observed my grandparents living very sedentary.

I had studied that many diseases were part and parcel of old age, but I observed that my grandparents had their shortcomings too. Being affluent and well-off, they could afford any food they desired. However, the disturbing part was their reluctance to exercise. Despite following healthy dietary habits, none of them made any worthwhile effort to lose weight. Though it had become crucial, both were reluctant to hit the gym or engage in exercises. Adding to their woes was that my grandfather was a heavy smoker who smoked about a packet of cigarettes daily. Since my junior education, this lifestyle invited my distrust because I had realized that engaging in an unhealthy habit, such as smoking, seriously affected a person's quality of life.

My grandpa's reluctance to visit a healthcare facility for regular check-ups aggravated the matter further. After some time, my grandpa started complaining of signs and symptoms that I later learned as a Registered Nurse related to kidney disease. These symptoms included muscle cramps, nausea, frequent vomiting, fatigue, and shortness of breath. He was referred to a dialysis unit for treatment. However, unfortunately, the persistent signs that were now being observed were an indicator of a much larger problem that had aggravated over a long time but had gone unobserved earlier. One day, following some time in the dialysis unit, I lost my grandpa.

I had performed hemodialysis treatment before my grandfather succumbed to exsanguination while undergoing dialysis. However, this tragedy shaped my future life. Being a registered nurse, I know how crucial dialysis is for treating kidney patients. Without routine dialyzing, patients—particularly the elderly and those with renal failure—can become lethargic, confused, bloated, and have skin thickness and color changes. They may find moving difficult due to fluid retention near their joints. Patients can and will suffer if a facility cannot meet their demands and fails to provide treatment even for a day or two. Death and excruciating anguish could be the end outcome.

Even though dialysis saves lives, the treatment procedure is marred by difficulties complicating this life-saving process. As a start, improving the health outcomes of the treatment requires both the patients and their families to demonstrate strength and resilience. Hemodialysis can be performed in a setting that is either an independent dialysis center or a facility that is a hospital division (referred to as a dialysis unit).

At the dialysis center, much time must be invested every week (about three times each week, for three to four hours per session). Therefore, adjusting to the hectic demands of dialysis could take time as patients eventually face the stark and challenging reality of aligning with the new norm in their lives. This novel experience is life-saving but requires consistency and a steadfast approach to ensure positive outcomes. Due to the challenges I experienced with my family after losing our grandpa. I developed a profound emotional attachment to helping improve patients' lives through Hemodialysis Regimen. However, frequent hemodialysis is essential for a kidney patient's body to maintain a healthy fluid and mineral balance and control blood pressure.

The sad part is that the dialysis treatment process is often marred by errors that can be avoided with education. I found this career very satisfying, with the role varying widely. Over time, I learned that my role as a renal nurse required being more than just a technical expert with a lot of knowledge and skills needed to simultaneously perform the roles of facilitator, mentor, caregiver, educator, and advocate. It is not just about providing dialysis therapy as ordered by the doctor. However, the role envisions a broader concept where I am bound to serve as an educator, advising patients on their illness, diet, medications, and other aspects. Most importantly, it is about working as a responsible team member and collaborating with the related staff to ensure compliance with treatment.

Starting my career as an R.N. at Chinatown Dialysis Center in N.Y., U.S., in 2009, the role of a qualified renal nurse with a nursing license has proven very rewarding. With its enormous demands, adjusting to the new position and setting, was challenging and disheartening to see your skills specified in one practice area. However, with time the role has proven very satisfying. Most importantly, renal nursing being a dynamic field, offers plenty of room for growth and improvement, albeit with its share of challenges.

An important aspect I observed in my experience working with patients was that I was required to work with patients in the long run.

This exposed me to one major challenge: I had to stay within professional boundaries while dispensing my responsibilities. It also meant striking the right balance in maintaining the relationship with patients and their families, who were now an essential part of my life, with many even regarding our team as an extended family. Ensuring patient compliance with the treatment protocol was another significant challenge as the patients were to be made aware of the need to comply with dietary, fluid, and medication regimens. The serious part about this role is that patients, at times, can be non-compliant, potentially threatening their lives with severe consequences such as hospitalization. Making the matter even more serious is the possibility that such non-compliance behaviors on the patients' part could even possibly lead to death.

Working on such a demanding schedule made me vulnerable to caregiver fatigue, as it was inevitable. The situation may take its toll on the patient's mental health as their lifestyle choices are increasingly restricted by their treatment protocol. However, the need of the hour was demonstrating patience and an informed approach to improve the lives of dialysis patients.

One of the exciting aspects of being a renal nurse is learning more about the patients. This typically requires every renal nurse to be essential to the patient's life. As I have known, creating an environment where everyone from the dialysis team to the patients and their families feels at home is important to improve treatment outcomes. I have found this approach effective in helping patients achieve the highest quality of life. Also, I found this approach highly rewarding because helping dialysis patients stay active and healthy instills an incredible feeling of accomplishment, knowing that your efforts were life-saving. In short, my career as a renal nurse was highly gratifying and boosted my self-esteem and satisfaction.

CHAPTER NINETEEN:
NXSTAGE HOME HEMODIALYSIS

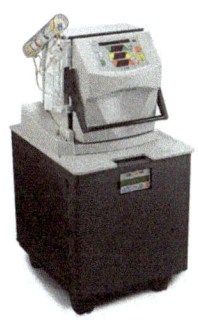

A brief overview of the NxStage machine and an Incenter dialysis

The NxStage refers to a home dialysis machine that acts as a traditional home alternative to dialysis. The NxStage machine can be incorporated into a home's setting with little changes required in the homes' electrical and plumbing.

An Incenter dialysis refers to a dialysis center where a kidney patient undergoes hemodialysis treatments.

Is Home dialysis better than in-center?

Home hemodialysis has some potential advantages over in-center dialysis. This treatment form will allow dialysis patients to schedule their treatments according to their routines. It allows the patient greater independence and more control of treatment. It also allows you the comfort and to be in the privacy of your own home.

NxStage System One S Home Machine operation mechanism

Being the first portable hemodialysis system that the FDA has specifically cleared, the machines and operation of the NxStage machine is easy to understand and follow. It is simple to use and has a revolutionary size of just about a foot tall. It allows the patients greater freedom to travel while performing the therapy.

Combined with the NxStage PureFlow SL Dialysis Preparation System, it involves a simplified process that requires ordinary tap water to serve as a dialysis fluid. NxStage machine enjoys an advantage over conventional hemodialysis systems because it requires no particular infrastructure.

NxStage is being used by the top hospitals across the U.S. the machine offers a broad range of flow rates which means the therapy can be individualized to the patients in the manner they choose. The machine is uniquely designed and offers a volumetric balancing system that ensures fluid accuracy without requiring scales. It eliminates the need for scale-based alarms. Interruptions caused by emptying waste bags unnecessary because the effluent flows into a space reserved as an open drain. It reduces staff workload because fluid accuracy is ensured without requiring scales.

The mechanism and operations of the NxStage involve no complex controls as its use is simple and intuitive, which paves the way for ease of use. User training is easy and simplified. It also requires no special electrical or plumbing services. Since the disposable cartridge is designed to ensure the elimination of blood-air interfaces, it helps reduce the risk of filter clotting.

Comparison and differences between Home Frequent Hemodialysis and Conventional thrice-weekly dialysis therapy

Home frequent hemodialysis offers considerable advantages to patients. Studies have concluded that this form of treatment leads to improved health outcomes. It promotes longer life and improves chances of survival if performed 5 to 7 times a week compared to conventional thrice-weekly dialysis therapy. It absolves the patients of the need to rely on a trained staff because the treatment can be performed without professional assistance after the patients have learned the process. Most importantly, this treatment is performed in the comfort of the home without requiring you to travel to a dialysis center. This option gives greater flexibility to the patients to choose a convenient time for performing dialysis. Patients feel better with a greater sense of control as they face fewer restrictions.

One of the main pressing issues with conventional thrice-weekly dialysis therapy is the significant change in fluid volume. In contrast, carrying out hemodialysis more often, such as home frequent hemodialysis, will reduce the common symptoms of kidney failure.

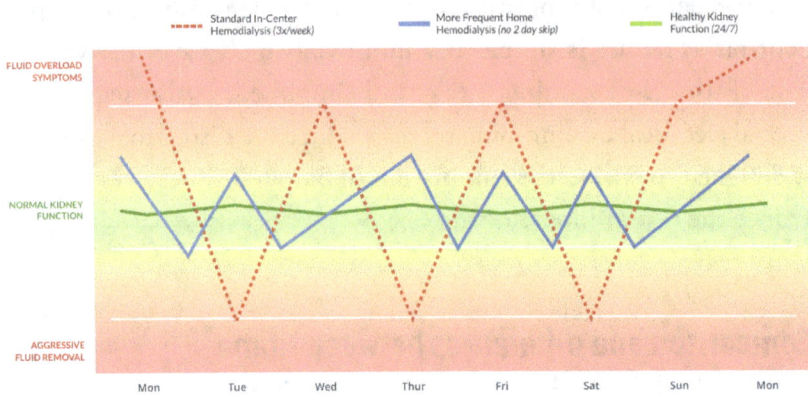

While there are significant advantages to each method, the critical part is that a kidney patient receives enough dialysis as it ensures an improvement in overall health. The right amount of dialysis will help patients feel better and keep them out of the hospital, besides letting them live longer. The doctor will decide on the 'dialysis prescription' to ensure the patient receives a sufficient treatment. It will depend on some factors, such as the fluid weight gained between the treatments, how well the kidneys are performing, body weight, and the waste present in the body.

The Advantages and Risks of Hemodialysis at In-Center /Skilled Nursing Facility

In-Center Hemodialysis is carried out in a dialysis center known as the in-center facility. This treatment takes place under the supervision of specially trained staff that is educated on delivering dialysis treatment. In this setting, the patient will need to visit the center thrice a week for treatment lasting between three to four hours.

Among the main advantages of in-center hemodialysis, patients can seek treatment overseen by trained professionals. It also allows the labs and patient assessment to be carried out at the hospital. The patients are in a better position to relax, read and socialize.

However, there are a few drawbacks as well. The patients would need to travel to the facility each time for treatment. The time must be adhered to as the timings may be inflexible and limiting. Since the treatment usually takes place thrice a week, the patients must adhere to a prescribed diet and limit fluid intake. Privacy in such a setting is not respected.

The Advantages and Risks of Hemodialysis at Home

There are many potential benefits of undergoing hemodialysis at home. The patients do not need to follow a strict schedule as they have greater flexibility in planning their treatment schedule. This, in turn, serves to boost overall mental health. With greater freedom to choose a dialysis schedule, it relieves mental stress. Also, not being required to travel to a center three times a week saves time. This treatment method can save up to 52 days per year for a dialysis patient in terms of time saved in recovery time, traveling, and waiting for appointments.

Studies have concluded that an increased number of treatments has other benefits too. It ensures a reduced reliance on medications. It also means an average of recovery, while the recovery time for in-center is at least eight hours. The improvement leading to better health levels allows such patients to be better positioned to receive a kidney transplant. It also puts the patient in control of their treatment.

Portable machines which are purpose-built for the home, such as NxStage System One, offer freedom to travel. This alleviates concerns about making alternative arrangements with dialysis centers away from your hometown.

There are also some risks associated with more frequent home hemodialysis. Though data indicates that such patients experience fewer complications and have improved clinical outcomes, certain risks that are prevalent in the home environment have also been identified.

Such treatments are performed without trained professionals' assistance or supervision of on-site technical support. Also, the vascular access obtained at home is exposed to more frequent use, which increases the chances of site infection and other related complications.

Reasons to choose the NxStage and Is it the Future of Home Hemodialysis?

There are many reasons to choose NxStage. It offers numerous advantages to those who want to make home hemodialysis a reality.

Most importantly, NxStage is a portable hemodialysis system. It comes with an interface that is easy to install and use at home. This machine offers great flexibility, making it easy to realize the dream of home hemodialysis. The machine has been designed for home patients because it offers a user interface for the patients.

The main advantage of this machine is that it allows frequent and flexible therapy at home. This means that the patients may schedule the treatment according to their choice. It allows the patient to enjoy more control and greater flexibility.

As mentioned above, the machine requires minor to no home renovations. This system also allows the patients to dialyze in any part of the home.

The machine is also designed for portability and can be moved around without hindrance or difficulty. Flexibility is also available when traveling as there are two methods of dialysate supply known as bags or Pure Flow SL.

The machine is also designed keeping in mind the ease of handling. It allows the treatment via a drop-in cartridge, making it easy. All that is required after treatment is removing the cartridge and wiping the device. Hence, the machine makes the dialysis process easy to perform. The drop-in cartridge offered by the NxStage machine includes an integrated dialyzer and bloodlines. This ensures an easy setup procedure. The cartridges are designed to reduce the risk of user errors that may otherwise be made on account of dealing with the dialyzer connections. It also reduces the risk of contamination which is a possibility when interacting with touch-point sites.

NxStage is the future of dialysis. It is the first portable hemodialysis system that has been cleared in the U.S. for home use. It includes solo hemodialysis (treatment performed during waking hours) and nocturnal hemodialysis (when the patient and caregiver can sleep).

NxStage has revolutionized dialysis treatment because it is designed to allow patients to benefit from this treatment at home. Since it is small and easy to carry, it offers patients greater freedom to travel.

CHAPTER TWENTY:
THE FUTURE OF YOUR HEALTH IS IN YOUR HANDS AND EVOLVING MODERN DIALYSIS TECHNOLOGY IS AROUND THE CORNER

Improvement in dialysis treatment outcomes

The past few years have been a game changer as the mortality rates for dialysis patients that showed no signs of declining for a significant part of the previous century witnessed a marked reduction. These declining mortality rates among maintenance dialysis patients were termed an outstanding achievement. However, despite this good news, there is still a strong need to build on these advances in care to sustain and increase survival gains.

A remarkable difference in the past decades for the medical field was that a reasonable sum of money was also invested in healthcare research along with the accelerating costs associated with medical care. The research proved very productive in terms of documenting and bringing about changes that boosted the quality and outcomes of care through the invention and innovation of the latest medical technology in the early years of the previous century,

Though much of the early attempts undertaken in managed care had offered limited effectiveness, it laid the foundation of a system that fostered care under the development of practice guidelines. The focus on the care delivery process has inevitably served to be a tremendous potential that can positively influence clinical practice with improved health outcomes.

The gloom surrounding dialysis treatment in the past is over

Statistics and figures, show that end-stage renal disease (ESRD) affects approximately 700,000 Americans. Of this affected population, around 400,000 have been put on life-saving hemodialysis therapy. Hemodialysis, despite being live-saving, has the potential to inflict a physical and emotional toll on hemodialysis patients. Unsurprisingly, most hemodialysis patients point out poor quality of life because they are put under this treatment. Regarding health-related quality of life (HrQOL), these patients have the worst outlook compared to patients afflicted with other chronic illness. This also includes those who have cancer and congestive heart failure. The poor quality of life faced by dialysis patients hurts their ability to manage their health. It affects self-care and usually results in poor health outcomes.

What the pandemic meant for dialysis treatment

The pandemic ushered in various habits that have become a norm in society. From wearing masks to focusing on hand washing, the world has readied itself and also embraced telehealth. Telehealth was heralded by the need to dodge the virus, leading to calls for shifting healthcare to home settings. This new concept now defines the world, and there is no going back, especially regarding dialysis therapy.

The importance of the home healthcare market cannot be underestimated, as this market was estimated to be worth a whopping $229 billion in 2020. With experts projecting its growth to accelerate by almost 8% annually, this new norm has revolutionized healthcare. Though some critics point out that the patients may have to lose some perks to avoid in-person interaction, this often translates to nothing. However, the benefits far outweigh the criticism as the patients gain the advantages of enjoying flexibility, control, and autonomy in benefiting from healthcare in the home setting.

This new norm is evident in all sectors of healthcare. The dialysis procedure regarded as too complex has also not remained unaffected by this change. Seeing others fare well without the need to travel to a hospital is now increasingly aligning to embrace the new methodology to avoid the hectic schedule that includes rigid clinic schedules and lengthy travel. This way offers a solution to the lengthy treatment periods and safety from the infectious environment the patients are exposed to in a healthcare setting. Most importantly, dialysis at home offers them a way to live fully as per their desires and wants. It is an expedient way for patients to take their health into their own hands.

Dialysis treatment has given new hope despite the need for further improvements

Despite the much skepticism surrounding dialysis treatment, it would be justifiable to state that this stems mainly from the need for further improvements in the treatment process rather than being an indicator that such treatment has not evolved to herald positive outcomes. The fact is that, as compared to the 1960s, kidney patients are living longer lives. They also lead more fulfilling lives with many choices available at their disposal. They have improved access to health care than their predecessors. However, there is no denying that more needs to be done. However, this need should include the significant accomplishments made over the recent decades in the dialysis treatment procedure.

Amidst all the gloom surrounding kidney disease, the good news for those 37 million Americans who live with kidney diseases and their families and loved ones is that the prospects of dialysis treatment have improved considerably over time. Kidney disease is a silent killer that inflicts its toll on patients, their families, and close ones. It also strains the healthcare system by consuming billions of healthcare costs. However, there is a need for immediate treatment because untreated kidney disease can potentially transform into an end-stage renal disease that requires dialysis or a transplant. Its progression can still be slowed down to a considerable extent by an intervention that includes effective treatment.

Though in the past, the first year of undergoing dialysis treatment was challenging for the patients due to the complex needs associated with this treatment. Nevertheless, the situation has improved with the number of patients suffering from kidney failure declining and those undergoing dialysis being able to live longer lives. In addition, less time now needs to be spent in hospitals. Overall, it has served to save lives and billions of dollars, allowing the healthcare system to invest in other directions.

Increased home dialysis will be the new norm in the future

Home dialysis is being dubbed the new norm, and rightly so, because it offers a convenient and effective solution to an ever-growing problem. Half a million Americans are already being treated with dialysis three times a week for four hours each session. Shifting the focus at home will be a welcome change. The current methods only increase the healthcare system's cost and add to the miseries of the patients.

Experts are constantly aiming to find better and safe ways that are proven efficient for dialysis treatment. There is also a need to ensure that dialysis providers are relieved of staffing and supply responsibilities. Along with these suggested barriers, plenty of others also need to be addressed and put in a system that would serve kidney patients most effectively while lowering the burden on the healthcare system.

The pandemic is another reason for the rising tendency to shift dialysis treatment to home. Avoiding Covid-19 is extremely important for kidney patients as they are vulnerable because they have a weakened immune system. Even if all precautions are to be practiced, a hospital setting will still expose kidney patients to more significant threat than at home. Staffing issues have intensified following the pandemic, prompting clinics to treat patients with fewer staff and spaces thereby magnifying the risks of Covid-19 infection manifolds.

Though figures suggest that almost 30% of dialysis patients are eligible for home dialysis, this advantage has yet to be utilized. Currently, only 2% of these patients receive treatment at home. Hence, making dialysis treatment available at home is the need of the hour.

What the future holds for dialysis treatment

Technological advancements and innovations are further expected to shape the future of dialysis treatment. All current dialysis methods are expected to become obsolete and only be replaced by more effective methods that provide improved health outcomes. It is also expected that smaller technology based on mobiles will be able to offer metabolic support. In the future, the devices are expected to be wearable or act as artificial kidneys that automate the body's metabolic functions.

All of this sounds like a dream, but this is a dream that is on its way to being realized on account of the advancements in science and technology. Mobile sensors that can collect necessary information, such as food intake and lifestyle habits, will also be a reality that will revolutionize kidney function and treatment. Furthermore, experts also suggest that there will soon be an integrated use of 3D-printed tissue and intelligent materials. These will serve as a replication for kidney design and function.

The ongoing research and success achieved make all these dreams exciting possibilities soon. It is yet to be ascertained what kidney treatment would be like in the next decade. However, it does hold the path to a healthier and more autonomous life for dialysis patients with a profound increase in survival rates.

INDEX

A

A fiber axon, 90
Acetate cellulose membrane dialyzer, 192
Acid reflux, 118
Acidic body, 118
Acidic pH, 118
Action potentials, 90
Acute Glomerulonephritis, 61, 63
Acute inflammation, 84
Acute kidney failure, 11, 12
Acute kidney injury (AKI), 21
Adaptive immune systems, 48
Aerobic pathogens, 80
Aerotolerant aerobes, 80
Albumin, 25
Albuminuria, 254
Alcohol, 28
Alkaline diet, 129
Alkalinizers, 145
Alpha-adrenergic agonists, 65
Altered mental status (AMS), 200
Alzheimer's, 77, 204
Amino acid hydroxyproline, 28
Amyloid angiopathy, 140
Anemia, 40
Aneurysms, 123, 164
Anemia, 23
Angiotensin II receptor blockers (ARBs), 65, 135
Angiotensin II, 2
Angiotensin-converting enzyme inhibitors (ACEIs), 65, 135
Angiotensinogenase, 4
Antibody test, 223
Anticoagulant drugs, 182
Antidiuretic hormone (ADH), 2
Antimicrobial peptide psoriasis, 47
Aranesp, 42, 44
Arterial clots, 141
Arterial gas embolism, 39
Arteriosclerosis, 120, 145
Arteriovenous fistula (AVF), 56, 150
Arteriovenous graft (AVG), 56, 150
Artificial additives and preservatives, 64
Artificial kidney machine, 63
Artificial Kidney, 190

Atherosclerosis, 123, 141
ATP production, 130
Autoimmune diseases, 82
Autoimmune disorder, 87
Autoinflammatory diseases, 87
Axon, 90

B

B2-microglobulin, 70
Baseline blood pressure, 32
Basic metabolic panel
    (BMP), 18
Behcet's disease, 87
Beta-adrenergic blockers. 65
Beta-amyloid, 77
Biomarkers, 83
Bladder infection (cystitis), 45
Blood clot (thrombus),
    107, 120
Blood electrolyte levels, 161
Blood flow rate (BFR), 20
Blood pressure (BP), 16, 131
Blood sugar, 98, 101
Blood urea nitrogen (BUN),
    16, 158
Blood viscosity, 101
Blood-brain barrier (BBB), 73
Blueberries, 5
Brain's monoaminergic
    system, 73
Butoconazole (Gynazole), 32

C

C fiber axons, 90, 91,
C-reactive protein (CRP), 74,
    75, 83
Calcification, 144
Calcinuria, 144
Calcitonin, 3
Calcitriol, 3
Calcium channel blockers, 65
Calcium homeostasis, 143
Cancer, 128, 129, 130
Candida infections, 32
Capillaries, 60
Cardiomyopathy, 143
Cardiovascular diseases,
    169, 170
Centers for Medicare &
    Medicaid Services
    (CMS), 234
Central line-associated
    bloodstream infections
    (CLABSIs), 29, 30
Central venous catheters
    (CVCs), 56, 57, 151
Chronic Glomerulonephritis, 63
Chronic Inflammation, 86
Chronic kidney disease
    (CKD), 11, 68
Chronic kidney failure
    (CKF), 11

Chronic traumatic brain injury (TBI), 42
Coagulase-negative, 29
Cognitive impairment, 71, 73
Collagen, 28
Collapsed lung, 40
Colonic microbiota 92
Comprehensive metabolic panel (CMP), 18
Communication skills, 259
Conditions for coverage (CfC), 214
Congestive heart failure, 142
Conventional home dialysis, 33
Cooling dialysate, 31, 115
Coronary artery disease, 175
Counseling, 207
Covid-19, 167, 279
CRBSI, 29
Creatinine clearance (CCr), 158
Creatinine, 156
Critical Thinking, 258
Cytokines, 75, 82

D

Deceased donor, 219
Deep vein thrombosis (DVT), 104, 107, 108
Dehydration, 8, 99, 100, 105, 106
Delirium, 204
Dementia, 202
Depression, 203
Deoxyribonucleic acid (DNA), 125
Dextran 40, 183
Diabetes, 45, 47
Diabetic ketoacidosis, 76
Diacetyl (Fearon), 17
Dialysate sodium prescription, 33
Dialysis prescription, 10
Dialysis Vintage, 172
Dialyzer, 190, 193
Diflucan (fluconazole), 32
Dihydroxyacetone (DHA), 92
Disequilibrium syndrome, 165
Diuretics, 64, 135
Drop-in cartridge, 273
Drug Abuse, 67
Dry Weight, 35, 36

E

Edema, 4, 84
Electrolyte imbalances, 10, 204
Elevated blood sugar levels, 201
Emphysematous cystitis, 47
End stage renal disease (ESRD), 156, 211
Endocarditis, 61
Enterococcus, 29
Enterohepatic circulation, 69
Enoxaparin, 182
Epinephrine, 182

Erythropoietin, 3, 4
Erythropoiesis-stimulating agents (ESAs), 43
Estimated glomerular filtration rate (eGFR), 2, 22

F

Facultative aerobes, 80
Fast pain, 90
Fatty acids, 53
Ferritin, 26
Fever, 78
Fibroblast growth factor (FGF23)phosphate, 73
Fight or flight, 196
Filamentous Fungus, 29
Filtration Fraction, 4
Flares (attack), 124
Fluid balance, 10, 37
Fluid overload, 10
Fluid volume, 38
Fructose, 20
Fungal growth, 34

G

Gangrene, 41, 123
Garlic, 5
Gastroesophageal reflux disease (GERD), 118, 119
Glomerular filtration rate (GFR), 72, 157, 212

Glomeruli, 60
Glomerulonephritis (GN), 59, 60, 61
Glucagon, 75, 76
Gluconeogenesis, 74, 75
Glycogenolysis, 75, 76
Glycosylated hemoglobin test (Hemoglobin A1c), 161
Gout, 125, 126
Gouty Arthritis, 128
Gram-negative organisms, 29
Gram-positive bacteria, 29
GT supplements, 32

H

Hand hygiene, 30
Heart attacks, 24, 141
Heartburn, 118, 119
Hematocrit, 159
Hemodialysis, 19, 33, 152, 153, 154
Hemeostasis management, 35
Hemodialysis, 19, 33, 152, 153, 154
Hemoglobin, 40, 159
Hemorrhagic stroke, 138
Heparin, 182
Hepatitis-related glomerulonephritis, 67
Heroin, 59
High blood sugar, 22
High flux dialysis, 70, 71

High fructose corn syrup (HFCS), 20, 127
High salt intake, 144
High sugar diet, 73
Hydration fluids, 100
Hydrogen peroxide, 92
Hyperbaric oxygen therapy (HBOT), 39
Hyperglycemia, 76, 77
Hypertension Diabetes, 18
Hypertension, 132, 133
Hyperuricemia, 124, 126
Hyperviscosity syndrome (HVS), 102
Hypervolemia, 10
Hypocoagulation, 103
Hypoglycemia, 76
Hypohydration, 105
Hypotension, 35
Hypoxia, 79, 80

I

Immune system, 47, 54, 167
Immunosuppressant drugs, 226
In-center hemodialysis, 33, 270
Indoxyl sulfate, 73
Industrial chemical, 87
Infections, 25, 41, 79, 87
Infective endocarditis, 41
Inflammation, 55, 81
Innate immune systems (Natural immune systems), 48

Insulin resistance, 106
Insulin, 47
Intra-dialytic hypotensive (IDH) episodes, 115
Intracranial hemorrhages, 138
Intravenous drug addicts, 67
Iron, 42
Ischemic strokes, 121

K

Ketoacidosis, 76
Kidney biopsy, 62
Kidney grafts, 230
Kidney recipients, 225, 226
Kidney Transplant, 219
Kidney-friendly diet, 6
Kidney, 1
KT/V, 19, 160

L

Lactate, 130
LDL, 250
Leafy greens, 53
Leptospermum scoparium, 91
Leukocyte, 85
Living donor, 219
Localized infection, 55
Low fat, 247
Low-acid diet, 129
Low-sugar diet, 32
Lupus, 59

M

Maintenance dialysis (MHD), 177
Maple syrup, 98
Marijuana, 59
Medicare Advantage Prescription Drug Plan, 237
Medium cut-off (MCO), 70
Mesenteric Ischemia, 121
Metabolic syndrome, 82
Metastasizing, 129
Methylglyoxal (MGO), 132
Microaerophiles, 80
Mircera, 44
Mood swings, 204
Mortality, 10, 167
Mucus, 50
Myelin, 90
Myoglobulin, 70

N

Natural blood thinners, 112
Necrotizing fasciitis, 41
Nephrons, 11, 22
Nephrotic syndrome, 66
Neurodegeneration, 73
Neuropsychiatric disorders, 71
Neutral pH level, 118
Neutrophils, 49
Nicotine, 59
Nociceptors, 87
Nocturnal home hemodialysis, 33, 273
Non-steroidal anti-inflammatory medicines, 183
Nucleic acids (ribonucleic acid), 125
Nxstage, 267

O

Obesity, 81, 122
Obligate aerobes, 80
Omega-3 fatty acids, 53
Onions, 5
Opine, 82
Osteomyelitis, 41
Oxalate, 28
Oxidative phosphorylation, 130

P

Pancreatic Failure, 24
Para-cresyl sulfate (PCS), 73
Pectin, 78, 79
Peptides, 53
Peripheral artery disease, 123
Peritoneal dialysis, 19
pH value, 2
Phagocytosis, 130
Phlegm, 50
Phlorotannins, 53
Phosphate binders, 27
Phosphorus, 7, 28

Plant-based diet, 27
Plaque, 122, 141
Plasma fibrinogen levels, 101
Plasma osmolality, 3
Plasma proteins, 102
Plasmapheresis, 64
Pluripotent stem cells, 24
Polycystic kidney disease, 220
Polysaccharides, 53
Potassium, 7, 162
Povidone-Iodine, 31
Preemptive kidney transplant, 222
Proinflammatory cytokines, 80
Protein C and S (Natural Anticoagulant), 110, 111
Protein-bound uremic toxins, 69
Protein, 7, 66, 75
Proteinuria, 15, 26
Psoriasis, 45
Psychiatric disorders, 72
Pulmonary edema, 141, 142
Pulmonary embolism, 108
Pus, 93
Pyelonephritis, 45

Q

Quality assessment and performance improvement process (QAPI), 212

R

Reactive oxygen species (ROS), 79
Red peppers, 6
Regenerated cellulose membrane dialyzer, 192
Renal abscesses, 47
Renal clearance, 3
Renal diet, 6
Renal vitamins, 53
Renin, 4
Replacing the fiber membrane dialyzer, 192
Rheumatoid Arthritis, 74

S

Sucrose, 20
Stem cell therapy. 24
Staphylococcus aureus, 29, 48, 49, 94
S. epidermidis, 49
Seaweeds, 53
Sepsis, 54
Systemic inflammation, 73, 75, 177
Systemic lupus erythematosus, 75
Symbiosis, 130
Shortness of breath (SOB), 44
Synthetic fiber membrane dialyzer, 192

Stress, 195
Subarachnoid hemorrhages, 139
Suicidal behavior, 204
Salt, 10, 131, 132
Serum creatinine level, 12

T

TCA cycle, 130
Terpenes, 53
Thrombocytopenia, 103
Thrombophilia, 104
Thrombosis, 104
Total urea clearance (KT/V), 155
Transient Ischemic Attack (KT/V), 123

U

Urea nitrogen, 18
Urea reduction ratio (URR), 160
Urea, 17
Uremia, 198
Uremic toxins, 177, 198
Uric acids, 124, 125
Urinary tract infections (UTI), 45

V

Vasopressin, 106

W

Water balance, 21
Water wise, 20
Water-soluble vitamins, 53
Water, 8, 46
White blood cells, 55
Whole grains, 5

www.ingramcontent.com/pod-product-compliance
Lightning Source LLC
LaVergne TN
LVHW021951060526
838201LV00049B/1663